COUNSELLING IDEOL

T0228261

It is easy to accept the heteronormative consciousness that informs and influences all aspects of psychotherapy. But it does not make it right. Queer theory offers radical insights into therapeutic logic and this book provides new and challenging perspectives on sex, gender and sexualities while giving language, communication, text and practice careful consideration. Questioning the process of therapy, this book offers ideas on reflection for practice and the development of theory in these areas.

Stephen Palmer, City University London, UK

Counselling Ideologies: Queer Challenges to Heteronormativity *offers a timely and significant interrogation of the transforming terrains of sexuality and psychology. The authors in this collection take up a number of critical questions concerning the constraints of heteronormative counselling ideologies on counselling practice and explore the expansive terrains of queer politics and queer theory to rethink both. The collection bridges theory and practice, drawing together insights from cultural studies of sexuality to refresh and reinvigorate the applied, professional dimensions of counselling and psychology. An excellent text.*

Deborah Lynn Steinberg, University of Warwick, USA

To my MC with all my love

Counselling Ideologies
Queer Challenges to Heteronormativity

Edited by

LYNDSEY MOON
University of Warwick, UK

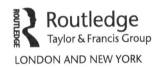

Routledge
Taylor & Francis Group

LONDON AND NEW YORK

First published 2010 by Ashgate Publishing

2 Park Square, Milton Park, Abingdon, Oxon OX14 4RN
711 Third Avenue, New York, NY 10017, USA

Routledge is an imprint of the Taylor & Francis Group, an informa business

First issued in paperback 2016

Copyright © 2010 Lyndsey Moon

Lyndsey Moon has asserted her right under the Copyright, Designs and Patents Act, 1988, to be identified as the editor of this work.

All rights reserved. No part of this book may be reprinted or reproduced or utilised in any form or by any electronic, mechanical, or other means, now known or hereafter invented, including photocopying and recording, or in any information storage or retrieval system, without permission in writing from the publishers.

Notice:
Product or corporate names may be trademarks or registered trademarks, and are used only for identification and explanation without intent to infringe.

British Library Cataloguing in Publication Data
Moon, Lyndsey, 1959-
   Counselling ideologies : queer challenges to
   heteronormativity.
   1. Sexual minorities--Psychology. 2. Sexual minorities--
   Counseling of. 3. Psychoanalysis and homosexuality.
   4. Heterosexism in medicine.
   I. Title
   616.8'917'0866-dc22

Library of Congress Cataloging-in-Publication Data
Counselling ideologies : queer challenges to heteronormativity / [edited] by Lyndsey Moon.
    p. cm.
   Includes index.
   ISBN 978-0-7546-7683-6 (hbk.) -- ISBN 978-0-7546-9361-1
(ebook) 1. Gays--Psychology. 2. Gays--Counseling of. 3. Sexual minorities--
Psychology. 4. Sexual minorities--Counseling of. 5. Queer theory--Psychological
aspects. 6. Psychotherapy. I. Moon, Lyndsey, 1959-
   RC451.4.G39C68 2009
   362.196'89008664--dc22

                                                                    2009052474

ISBN 13: 978-0-7546-7683-6 (hbk)
ISBN 13: 978-1-138-26028-3 (pbk)

Contents

Acknowledgements

I have quite a number of people to thank for being alongside at different stages in the writing of this book. It has been a tough challenge at times and I want to thank Neil Jordan at Ashgate for putting faith in the book. I want to give a big thank you to all those who offered their time and efforts to each chapter because without them, this book simply would not exist. In particular, I would like to thank Professor Deborah Lynn Steinberg who has been encouraging and steadfast and is always an inspiration. I would like to thank the Sociology Department at Warwick for generously offering me the space and time to enjoy participating in debate – both serious and fun – which offered plenty of new ideas. I would like to say thanks to Roz and Trill who I love dearly. I want to thank my partner, Lal, for her patience and resilience – especially in those late night hours. Finally, I want to thank my mum and dad who I treasure. All three of us share in the deeply tragic loss of my brother, Guy, who we continue to miss and will always be a precious part of my life.

List of Contributors

Y. Gavriel Ansara (席嘉力 /ﺗﺂﺷ ﺟﻭﺍﺩﻳ/ﺑﺮﻳﺎﻟﺃ ﻳﺮﺴﺗ) earned his MSc with Distinction in Social Psychology from the University of Surrey, where his current PhD research on cisgenderism is funded by a departmental bursary. Gavi recently joined The Kerulos Centre as Teaching Faculty involved in curriculum development and is co-author of a chapter on gender identity/expression and bullying in *Bully-Proofing Your School: Cultural Proficiency* (forthcoming), with child psychologist Carla Garrity of the Neuro-Developmental Ctr (Denver, CO). During a sojourn in the US, his pioneering work as founder and coordinator of the Tiferet Outreach Project earned him the Keshet 2002 Leadership of the Year Award. From 2006–2008, he founded and directed Lifelines Rhode Island/Cuerdas de Salvamento, a state-wide advocacy, education, and support organisation serving individuals of trans, non-binary gender, and intersex experience, and was subsequently awarded the 2008 Lifelines Pillar of the Community Award by board members and volunteers. He is UK Speaker on Multicultural Issues for Organisation Intersex Internationale and the first elected Trans Representative Officer of Surrey's LGBT Society. As a polycultural Empath and Healer with a multinational background and heritage, he is committed to Tikkun Olam (improving the world and establishing sanctity within it).

Sekneh Beckett is coloured by her Lebanese Muslim ancestry. She is a registered Psychologist and Narrative Therapist. Sekneh maintains a private practice in Sydney providing counselling, consultancy, supervision, and teaches for the Dulwich Centre (Adelaide), and the Postgraduate Social Health and Applied Psychology Course at Macquarie University. Her community work in the GLBTIQ communities has been recognised and in 2004 she was awarded the Community Supporter of the Year. She enjoys re-searching peoples creative ways of being in the world, and engaging with the politics of therapeutic and community work. Sekneh can be contacted via sekbeckett@hotmail.com.

Catherine Butler works as a principle clinical psychologist, trainer and systemic psychotherapist in Hackney Primary Care Trust. Prior to her work in adult mental health with this trust, she worked in NHS sexual health services in central and south London for five and a half years. During this time she developed a couples' service, a HIV training program for African Communities, and provided national training on working with lesbian and gay clients and 'Motivational Interviewing'. She was the research officer on the BPS HIV and Sexual Health Faculty committee, where her work included organising national conferences, writing national guidelines, conducting audits and publishing articles. Her research interests include sexual assault, the use of interpreters, and the personal and professional integration of lesbian and gay psychologists. Catherine has also worked in the private and voluntary sector, including as a couple/family therapist at PACE and as a therapist, trainer and Clinical Associate with Pink Therapy. She was previously on the BPS Lesbian and Gay Psychology Subsection committee and won their postgraduate research prize.

Mark Casey is a Lecturer in Sociology at Newcastle University where he teaches in the areas of sexuality, gender and tourism. He is currently involved in a research project with Dr Yvette Taylor and Michelle Addison examining the everyday lives of lesbian and gay men in the North East of England. He has recently been writing around gay male identity, travel and sex, publishing in *Leisure Studies* (2009) 'Toursit Gay(ze) or Transnational Sex: Gay Men's Holiday Desires' and has the chapter 'Even Poor Gays Travel: Excluding Low Income Gay Men from Understandings of Gay Tourism' in Taylors (2010) edited collection *Classed Intersections: Spaces, Selves, Knowledge.* Mark has a growing interest in the intersection between sociological understandings to gay men's identities and approaches used by those working in mental health. He has published on this topic recently with the paper 'Addressing Key Theoretical Approaches to Gay Male Sexual Identity: Issues and Insights for Practitioners' in the journal *Critical Public Health* (2009) and in this volume. He is currently editing, along with colleagues, a special edition of *Sociology* (2010) on sexualities.

Dossie Easton is a Marriage and Family Therapist in private practice in San Francisco since 1991, a certified supervisor of interns in training and a continuing education provider offering classes to other professionals working with lifestyle minorities. She has worked in the BDSM communities since 1973, and is familiar with how S/M people form relationships, make provisions for consent and safety, and deal with the emotional consequences of playing with power. She is co-author with Janet W. Hardy of four books dealing with various aspects of S/M lifestyles, and a fifth on polyamorous relationships.

Ian Hodges is a Senior Lecturer in Psychology at the University of Westminster. He teaches in the following areas; psychotherapy and counselling, critical psychology, psychology of prejudice, and qualitative methods. His research interests include; using psychoanalytic approaches with sexual minority clients, challenging heteronormativity in psychoanalytic theory and practice, queer theory, and psychotherapeutic discourse. He is currently training at the Site for Contemporary Psychoanalysis.

Alessandra (Alex) Iantaffi received a PhD from the University of Reading (UK), and a MSc in Systemic Psychotherapy from the University of Bedfordshire (UK) after moving from Italy to the UK in 1993. Alex's research interests and publications have focused on gender, higher education, disability, sexuality, polyamory and BDSM. She is also the editor of the international *Journal of Sexual and Relationship Therapy* and is currently working at the Program in Human Sexuality at the University of Minnesota (USA). Email: ianta001@umn.edu.

Christian Klesse is Senior Lecturer in Cultural Studies at the Department of Sociology at Manchester Metropolitan University. He has published widely on sexuality, intimacy, body modification, sexual politics and research methodology. He is author of *The Spectre of Promiscuity: Gay Male and Bisexual Non-Monogamies and Polyamories* (Ashgate 2007). He is currently undertaking research together with Jon Binnie (also MMU) into transnational activism regarding LGBTQ politics in Poland.

Tina Livingstone is a Client Centred Therapist based in Southampton. She has been involved with the trans community since 1990 and provides online support for Transsexual and Intersex people. She welcomes all clients with genuine respect and equanimity. Tina is at ease with the natural diversity of sexual orientation, respecting relationships both within and outside of traditional partnerships. She has successfully delivered 'Awareness Raising' workshops and presentations concerning matters such as Gender Transition, Intersex Issues, Civil Rights and Welcoming Diversity.

Lyndsey Moon, PhD, is a Senior Lecturer at Roehampton University where she lectures in Counselling Psychology, and held an ESRC funded Senior Research Fellowship in the Department of Sociology at Warwick University at the time of writing. She published *Feeling Queer or Queer Feelings: Radical Approaches to Counselling Sex, Gender and Sexualities* published by Routledge in 2007. She has also worked in the field of alcohol and drugs for the past 20 years. She researches sex, genders and sexualities and their relationship to counselling psychology and psychotherapy. Email: lyndsey.moon@roehampton.ac.uk or L.Moon@warwick.ac.uk.

Roshan das Nair works as a Consultant Psychologist in HIV and Sexual Health with the Department of Clinical Psychology and Neuropsychology at the Nottingham University Hospitals NHS Trust, and as a Research Tutor on the Trent Doctorate in Clinical Psychology programme at the University of Nottingham. He has previously worked in the areas of sex, sexuality, and HIV/AIDS in Zambia and India. Roshan is a Board Member of the Nottingham Sexual Health Providers' forum. He is the Editor-in-chief of the *Psychology of Sexualities Review* of the British Psychological Society's (BPS) Psychology of Sexualities Section. He is also their representative on 'The International Network on Lesbian, Gay, and Bisexual Concerns and Transgender Issues in Psychology'. He has been a member of the Working Party responsible for writing the BPS guidelines on 'Working Therapeutically with Sexual and Gender Minority Clients'.

David Nylund, PhD, MSW, is an Associate Professor of Social Work at California State University, Sacramento, and a clinical supervisor at La Familia Counseling Services and the Sacramento Gay and Lesbian Center. David is the co-editor (with Craig Smith) of *Narrative Therapies with Children and Adolescent* and the author of *Treating Huckleberry Finn: A New Narrative Approach with Kids Diagnosed ADD/ADHD*. His latest book is *Beer, Babes, and Balls: Masculinity and Sports Talk Radio*, and is published by SUNY Press.

Sonya Thomas works as a freelance writer and equality consultant and has over 20 years' experience of equalities work, both in the public and voluntary sectors. She has provided political advice on equalities to local government elected members and political leads and has authored a number of speeches on various aspects of equalities and diversity for Commissioners within the Equality and Human Rights Commission and senior civil servants in the Department of Health.

Julie Tilsen, MA, is a therapist, consultant and trainer noted for her breadth and depth of clinical experience. She provides training and consultation to a variety of youth-serving and community-based agencies. Julie is a licensed Psychologist in Minnesota and a registered Clinical Counselor in British Columbia, and holds a MA in Counseling Psychology from Saint Mary's University in Minneapolis.

PART I
De/Heterosexualising Therapy

Introduction

Lyndsey Moon

Queer Causes Trouble

I am looking at a photo emblazoned: 'The Front banner of the Yellow Queer Feminist Block'. It is a banner several feet long and high, so high that all we can see are a row of heads from those people behind and their fists tightly holding the banner in a long row across the top. It is being held up by queers of all ages, colours and abilities who are on a march with many others through the streets of a major European City. To the right side of the banner it shows a sign of a large fist smashing through what looks like an image of glass and there are symbols of shards of glass occupying the space around the fist, while to the left of the fist, are the words 'Normalize This' with star signs around it – almost parodying the words. The photo is striking because of its simplicity, its audacity, its resistance and its power. The fist is aimed at 'you', and it is being carried en force by many hundreds of followers who are marching forward over the time worn tarmac laid down by a past generation. 'You' represent a force that may only be responded to through a queer stance that demands attention and respect. Queer elucidates a social subjectivity that is determined to challenge assimilation and embrace fear. The 'normal' people are gradually being pushed to the fringes and stand to each side – people looking with apprehension and bewilderment at this vivid spectacle, this movement of future in their present. It feels uneasy. There is a tension, a slight sigh of breath as I gaze upon what this image means while at the same time the vision is contesting my own thoughts and ideas. It is a vision that refuses to compromise, refuses to assimilate and generates a critical interrogation of the taken for granted notion of what constitutes 'normality'. It is for this latter reason that I have introduced this picture, this rather contentious image. It marks a turning point, a critical edge, a new perspective that therapeutic ideology needs to grab hold of and take into account. It is no longer acceptable to look at the therapies through heterosexual signification – through those processes of meaning-making which fail to disturb heterosexual representations. It is time for change.

Queer theory means unsettling conventional therapeutic theories and practices while it transforms understandings of, and approaches towards, sex, genders and sexualities. It seems an odd and somewhat problematic statement to suggest that therapy needs a social and 'queer' theory to act as a transformative potential in re-shaping practices and ideological stance. But this is implicitly or explicitly recommended throughout the chapters. Sexual agency in relation to therapeutic

structures is brought under scrutiny in order that it severely disrupts the taken for
granted heteronormative consciousness that pervades all therapeutic structures.
Instead, a queer consciousness is considered and commented upon. The first four
chapters take up this slogan by declaring the de/heterosexualisation of therapy.
The following seven chapters show how this may be operationalised through
resistance and contestation. They highlight ways in which queer theory can
decentralise therapeutic ideology and normative thinking in relation to issues such
as queer spaces, bisexuality, non-monogamy, BDSM, cisgenderism, working with
Muslim gay men, race and gender.

The first part presents the case for de/heterosexualising therapy and opens
with chapters that focus on the way therapy is embedded within heteronormative
and regulatory discourses that 'discipline' personhood. They question the very
structural composition of therapy. The chapters open with Tina Livingstone's
contribution to thinking about regulatory discourses, how sex is linked to 'talk'
that is 'dirty' and how it is time to unpack the dictionary of words therapy is
built upon such as 'disorder' and 'defect', how these become naturalised and
internalised. Alternatively, Tina points out that some clients want to conform to
'normality', want to feel accepted by a normative society and, as they are already
deeply sanctioned against because of their gender and/or sexuality, they no longer
want to transgress, they simply want to find their place in life. She introduces
the idea of cisgenderism, a theme later written about by Gavriel Ansara, where
personhood is based on gender being aligned to designated biological sex and
yet this is now so limiting that it must change or continue to fracture the whole
meaning of personhood. The question is how therapists can work with such a
limiting concept? How can therapists work with meanings of 'authenticity' and
'congruency' when their own understanding is incongruent with social meanings?
For example, how do therapists respond to the idea that as a child, their client may
have dressed in clothing designed for the opposite gender – what does this mean? If
the social narratives were such that 'dressing-up' in all shapes of 'identity' clothing
was normative then how would the meanings of gendered childhood development
change? It is this type of thinking that needs to shift – particularly for therapists.
As Tina states, 'queer isn't about the people it's about the process' which is the
basis on which this and the following chapters are written.

In Chapter 2, Ian Hodges argues for a queer re-reading of classical psychoanalysis
through Butler, Kristeva and Derrida and remarks upon the constant ambivalence
and contradiction towards queer sexualities within the psychoanalytic landscape.
Ian brings into focus the meaning of the Oedipus complex and questions what
would happen to this representational model if Western social power relations
and values were dismantled in relation to gender and sexuality. In Chapter 3, Alex
Iantaffi extends the idea of therapy as a social process and the way reflexivity
is central to training. She scrutinises epistemological shallowness and wants to
create new narratives that usurp heterosexual dogma. We read about the tensions
inherent within training regimes and the way 'curiosity' is vanquished within
heteronormative training. This notion of curiosity is a theme that needs to be played

with in therapy and Alex shows how research and training need to be inquisitive, questioning and enquiring if they are to integrate new meanings for experiences. In Chapter 4, I write in relation to feeling and emotion and suggest that desire and feeling need to be freed from the materiality of the body seen as 'identity'. Although useful in the past, my argument suggests that identity as a structure is now limiting and rather than freeing desire, it now constrains sexual feelings towards the 'other'. Looking towards queer as a form of praxis as well as theory, I argue that queer is gradually dismantling present representations of desire and forming new meanings for bodies that are no longer limited by identities.

In Part II, the focus moves to relations of resistance and contestation. Starting with Chapter 5, Julie Tilsen and David Nylund, question the generational discourses, the shifts in meaning for queer youth and the concept of heteronormativity as a result of 'neo-liberal and assimilationist identity politics'. Throughout the chapter they promote the use of discursive therapy practices informed by poststructuralist thinking and bring about a disruption of conventional therapeutic narratives. They insert the idea of 'reverse discourse' and how this may be used to change, rather than overturn, the meaning of power. Drawing from shared narratives with queer youth, they see these as transgressive stories of revolution in everyday life.

Following on from this, in Chapter 6, Catherine Butler, Roshan das Nair and Sonya Thomas present a discursive account of queer theory in relation to 'people of colour', arguing that queer remains 'black and white'. Presenting a 'white queer theory' where they argue that queer theory is shaped by a 'white perspective' they follow this with a 'black queer theory' which provides a way of collating the history and practice of writing about black, colour and queer that therapists need to engage with in terms of a critical thinking style. In sum, they provoke ideas and suggest the reader further analyses race and its interaction with queer theory.

In Chapter 7, Christian Klesse introduces bisexuality, challenging the manner in which non-heterosexual forms of intimacy become legitimated through monogamy. He shows how counselling and therapy struggle with meanings about bisexuality both theoretically and for client work and he introduces ideas for therapists to consider when faced with bisexual issues such as non-monogamy, bi-phobia, bi-negativity, kinship structures and polyamoury.

Chapter 8 finds Mark Casey presenting his work in relation to lesbians, gay men and queers in the north east of England. Alongside debates that surface in relation to 'issues' such as queer geographical locations and scene space, Mark tackles how therapists conducting research need to be reminded about the reasons for collecting demographic details and how these impact on the meaning of client narratives when age, race, ability, ethnicity, sexuality, gender and sex are all constantly interacting. He shows how, if research is not thorough in its collection of material, then the application of results are limited and limiting. But Mark also interrogates the meaning for therapy of queer spaces and how these position the individual within a complex set of representations. For example, home life is central to our experience of socialisation while age is a factor in constant need of evaluation and scene spaces are always in need of interrogation. Using sociological analyses, both Christian and Mark offer new insights into the meaning of social issues and show their relevance to everyday social and personal life meanings.

The final three chapters again offer insights into therapeutic areas we rarely acknowledge: cisgenderism, Muslims who are negotiating their sexual identity and the role of power in therapy as shown by the practice of BDSM and understanding this through psychodynamic theory.

In Chapter 9, cisgenderism is Gavi Ansari's main focus where he shows the basic inadequacy of therapeutic meanings for trans experiences. He acknowledges political issues of funding and how this leads to an 'alphabet soup' approach to ways of understanding trans people whereby there is an implicit assumption that all trans people are the 'same'. It introduces the idea of lack of recognition and calls upon ways that change may be brought about through a 'social justice activism' whereby therapy no longer disguises or shies away from its political sensibilities, but actively engages with a democratising and liberatory agenda to the benefit of all clients.

In Chapter 10, Sekneh Beckett writes about her work with Muslim clients negotiating their sexual identity and the 'games of truth' that emerge when discourses are made transparent. She focuses on the myths that are made material and put to rest on both the individual and social body.

Finally, Chapter 11 by Dossie Easton, provides the backdrop to sado-masochistic practices, bondage and domination and how these may be used positively within therapeutic discourse with clients who present as wanting to explore sexual meanings and drama in order to develop their personal sexual story.

In conclusion, I do believe that each chapter acts as a queer narrative revealing ways that can benefit therapeutic discourse and practice. More importantly, it shifts meanings, representations and discourses in relation to dissident sex, sexualities and genders to the forefront of social change. Therefore, I take this opportunity to thank all those who have contributed towards the disruption of heteronormativity and hope that those reading the text take up the challenge to criticise therapeutic narratives that are embedded within a normative framework.

Chapter 1

Anti-Sectarian, Queer, Client-Centredness: A Re-Iteration of Respect in Therapy

Tina Livingstone

Context

The extent of regulatory discourse applied to relationships and 'rude bits' shows that, for a sexually reproductive social species, we seem to have inordinate difficulty with these fundamental aspects of our existence. Despite the bold titling of theatrical productions such as 'The Vagina Monologues' (Ensler 2007) and 'Puppetry of the Penis' (Morley and Friend 2000) characteristic use of euphemism for sexual body parts and sexual acts persists in modern culture; the 'covering' of words mirroring the covering of sexual shame. A mix of statutory legislation and cultural norms strongly impact on how our sex and sexuality is understood and 'done'. Zerubavel (2006, 27–28) notes 'the under-lying assumption behind the social taboo on the use of various sex-related ("dirty") words is that it is quite possible to actually eliminate certain ideas by sanitizing our discourse'. Constraints on gender identity and expression prove even more strenuous; as Jay notes 'tabooed thoughts remain taboo because there is no acceptable way to depreciate them through public discussion' (1999, 128). The lack of a common vocabulary beyond binarian gender terms is then a strong indicator of how unacceptable it is to be beyond those norms.

Society polices sex, sexuality and gender with such rigidity that people who appear to flout heteronormative constructs confound to the extent that they are viewed at best sceptically and often with fear. Those who appear to transgress these norms in any way are persistently deemed defective, disordered and dangerous by our most powerful regulatory triad – religious, secular and medical discourse. Heterosexist discourse problematizes gender diversity similarly to homosexuality 'as a sin (in religious discourse); as unnatural (in both religious and secular discourse); as an illness (in medicine and psychiatry …); as a congenital disorder or inversion (in sex psychology and sexology); as deviance (in some sociological theory); … as child molesters, seducers, and corruptors (in certain sexological studies, the law and the media)' (Kinsman 2006, 103). Society is not simply hierarchically segregated with regard to gender diversity, it has become sectarian. One of the most profound methods of social control is to label something deviant – thus providing 'a clear-cut, publicized, and recognizable threshold between permissible and impermissible behaviour' serving 'to segregate the deviants from others' (McIntosh 2001, 426).

Socio-medical discourse has always had fundamental connections with the principle of social control, indoctrinated by the premise that if an aspect of humanity deviates from the norm, it needs to be cured or 'cut off', i.e. removed surgically or psychologically. Psychiatry expanded this hegemony by conflating the notion of being 'mentally ill' with 'dangerous', a fusion that remains inextricably linked for many even in contemporary society. This perception of sameness arises from the fact that historically society did not differentiate between outcasts: the poor, prostitutes, criminals, the infirm and those regarded morally defective or insane were all confined to the same places – the mad-, poor-, work-houses or gaol. The concept of commonality between populations deemed 'mad, sad, and bad' is then culturally based, and socially constructed regulative discourse is devilishly hard to shift. We are still working with a good deal of residual fear from this diagnosis of dangerous on both sides.

Krafft-Ebing's view of 'antipathic sexuality' as an 'abnormal manifestation' of varying degrees – roughly corresponding to our present day categories of bisexual, homosexual, transsexual and intersex – was transparent in its heteronormative morality:

> Untainted man will never become sexually inverted through onanism or seduction by persons of the same sex; for as soon as the extrinsic influences cease he returns to normal sexual functions. The tainted individual, however, whose psycho-sexual centre is originally weak, is in a different position ... evil influences may render him furthermost psychically bisexual, then invertedly mono-sexual, and eventually may even effect castration. (1886, 230)

Over a century later persistent notions of psychological fault and weakness are shown by the continuance of sex and gender diversity in both DSM IV TR[1] and ICD-10.[2] The realm of the helping professional is not yet without concepts that collude with the premise that sexual and gender variations arise from defect and disorder. Preoccupation with the naturalness of perceived binaries also propagates the disordering of bodies beyond accepted pattern. Whilst the intersex population were not so directly psycho-pathologized, Krafft-Ebing's note that 'Gynecomastia only occurs in neurotically degenerated families' (1886, 29), provides some insight into the socio-medical discourse that pressured the families concerned into sustaining secrecy through shame. Since biological division of the sexes actually rests on gamete size, the best we can actually say is that in *most* cases

---

1   See *Diagnostic and Statistical Manual of Mental Disorders 4th Edition*, 2000, pp. 576–582, Washington, American Psychiatric Association.

2   See *International Statistical Classification of Diseases and Related Health Problems 10th Revision*, Version for 2007, Disorders of adult personality and behaviour (F60-F69), World Health Organization <http://apps.who.int/classifications/apps/icd/icd10online/>.

human beings are biologically configured in one of two general patterns – labelled male and female. All other indicators being variable, the universal application of binary reductionism proves as problematic in anatomy as psychology. Being born intersex remains so heavily sanctioned that those not directly affected often remain blissfully unaware that such situations even exist, and for the sake of conformity families may still be encouraged to accept the surgical alteration of their offspring in infancy as social necessity. Aside from the fact such procedures are rarely singular, often leading to physical scarring and sexual dysfunction, my experience as counsellor informs me that this process frequently leaves intersex people with the excruciatingly painful notion that they are intrinsically unlovable. A poignant illustration of the continued sectarianizing of sex non-conformity, profoundly affecting the lives of both intersexual and transsexual people, can be found in Feinberg's encounter with a doctor when sie (gender neutral pronoun pronounced 'see') was seriously ill with endocarditis:

> When he determined that my anatomy was female he flashed a mean spirited smirk … He ordered me to leave the hospital and never return. I refused. I told him I wouldn't leave until he could tell me why my fever was so high. He said "You have a fever because you are a troubled person". (1998, 2)

Humankind has always been intrigued by the mysteries of life, but whilst the intangibles of inner self and attraction are understandably open to curiosity, it is blatantly tyrannical to label those who do not fit cultural norms as defective and disordered. This situation is most disturbing – profoundly so for many of my clients; in a relational world they feel excluded from relating, consequently spending considerable time contemplating the whys and wherefores, and striving to reconcile the situation.

Summary of Threads

'Queer' is a word most of my minorities' clients would not hold comfortably, in fact many would wonder what I am doing writing here. As an umbrella term for non-normative sexual identities 'queer' implies a radical anti-assimilationist stance, asserting an 'in-your-face difference, with an edge of defiant separatism' (Gamson 2001, 521). Since many of my clients' existences already fall outside conventional social markers relating to gender, sex and sexuality, to such extent they are alienated, they are understandably anxious of any further separation. Identities deeply sanctioned and constrained by social discourse and its regulatory practices put people on the edge of existence, and so much as edges can feel exciting, most of us do not want to sit on one all the time. Most clients do not come to therapy seeking to transgress social norms – they come to find a sense of place in the world through an understanding of their experiences and how this relates to ideas of selfhood, to recover from personal traumas, and with life struggles that they wish to resolve – a space where they can begin to unpack the meaning of what is happening in life. Most do not wish to walk on the wild side, exist in some sexual twilight zone, nor provide some epitome of political principles; consequently the 'queer' in my therapy does not so much concern the nature of the people but the principles and practice of the process.

Initially trained in the 'Client Centred' approach, I would still regard myself as closely aligned to that model; despite the way queer may challenge subjectivity, and what this means, some clients do want to explore who they are in the social world and what it means for them. I believe the most effective therapeutic alliance is underpinned by unconditional positive regard for the client, built on congruence, and enabled by the striving for, and communication of, empathic understanding. Queering that process is about consciously enabling the client to engage in less marginalized and oppressive spaces through genuine respect for autonomy. Avoidance of odious labels and resistance to any 'a priori' agenda, however well intentioned, is paramount in the co-construction of less constricting subjectivities. It is not my responsibility to set the route or destination – but to be alongside the client on his/her/hir journey, enabling the discovery and engagement of skills necessary for that client to live more comfortably.

Working in the main with trans-identified, trans-historied and intersex populations I am acutely aware of the sectarianism that not only divides them from the heteronormative mainstream, but also from the sexual minorities with whom they have become associated, and indeed within their own populations. My understanding of sectarianism is that it exists within cultural commonality, and comprises factions set against each other by reason of doctrine and dogma. Originally ascribed to religion, it is no stranger to the political, secular or medical realms. Shirley recognized that secular sectarianism was 'quite as detrimental to freedom of heart and breadth of intellect' as religious sectarianism in the nineteenth century and observed 'The spirit of persecution is just the spirit of exclusiveness, under another and more aggressive aspect' (1859, 444). Unfortunately this spirit remains alive and well in the realms of sex and gender, and is particularly acute with regard to trans' and intersex identities.

As Leary observes 'We know that not everyone will necessarily like us, but we usually hope that they will at least not find us so deficient or aversive as social interactants that they reject us outright' (2001, 3). Social stigma and the sectarianism it propagates does much to defeat that hope. What follows concerns my perceptions of three degrees of separation experienced by the transgendered population how those may impact the client, and some of the principles and practise I employ in helping my clients work through them.

First Separation

It seems inherent to construct boundaries; our quest for order is so insatiable that where they don't exist we will build them. Concepts of *infinite* and *limitless* do not sit well with ritualistic creatures who strive to make sense of everything so it is containable. Reduction makes things manageable and, simple creatures that we are, our favourite number is two. Day and night, up and down, this and that, man and woman – everything not only has a place, it can be reduced to a binary. Moreover as social animals who thrive on hierarchy everything is ranked – there is always a top and a bottom (switching is just too sassy). The present constructs of male and female, and resulting binary of masculinities and femininities, are then so rigid that they effectively exclude those who experience themselves differently, whether within that binary or beyond it.

Within such sectarian climate 'Both the individuality of humans and their membership in the universal category of humanity are rejected or downplayed in favour of these specific categories of identity' (Good 2001, 22); creating a situation where the person is all too often lost under their label. Good notes that if people 'are not treated primarily as individuals but as representatives of their demographic category, their dignity and autonomy are diminished' (2001, 27). Our culture is not simply heterosexually biased, being cisgendered (having psychological gender aligned with biological sex) underpins that norm and is thus culturally embedded to such an extent that those experiencing themselves differently gendered frequently feel their claim on the word 'person' itself denied. This was pragmatically explained to me some years ago by a friend who noted 'Just as I am not "A Blind" so I am not "A Transsexual"; I am a person who happens to be both partially sighted and transsexual'. Accepting the first necessary and sufficient condition for effective therapy as 'Two *persons* (my emphasis) are in psychological contact' (Rogers 1989, 221), it feels fundamentally important to recognize that many gender variant clients feel their claim on personhood itself denied, and consequently work to restore it. Where otherness in sex and gender has been ascribed either abnormal or abhorrent, rejection and ridicule are not only par for the course but sometimes taken as inevitable consequence on both sides. This de-humanizing of human beings within the context of sex and gender variation is evidenced by the frequent emergence of the question '*What* am I?' in therapy. Whereas Rogers entered his therapy sessions with the question 'How can I provide a relationship which this person may use for his own personal growth?' (1961, 32), I often find myself feeling a step back from that, wondering 'How can I provide a relationship within which this individual may come to an understanding of themselves as a valid person?' This is no glib concern: when people feel their authenticity as human beings fundamentally challenged it is sectarianism at its most iniquitous. Mearns and Thorn have observed that:

> all too many of those who seek the help of counsellors have spent much of their lives surrounded by people who, with devastating inappropriateness, have appointed themselves experts in the conduct of other people's lives. As a result such clients are in despair at their inability to fulfil the expectations of others, whether parents, teachers, colleagues or so-called friends, and have no sense of self respect or personal worth. (2007, 10)

Those clients whose basic identity has been the subject of (and possibly totally ascribed by) outside agencies sometimes find it hard to recognize themselves as persons at all, let alone grasp any wisp of personal worth. There is a marked difference between ones preferences and behaviours being regarded as undesirable, even unnatural, and being fundamentally denied as a person. Facilitating positive therapeutic change sometimes first needs to co-construct the validity of my client as person: a fragile concept for those who have accepted configurations of trans-identity or intersex as the sum of their existence rather than aspects of self. Facilitating somebody's discovery of their own humanity can be a precarious process since one could easily violate the client's autonomy by setting oneself up as judge, caretaker or expert, rather than therapist. This comprises carefully removing the blinkers created by judgement laden labels, enabling non-judgmental identification of this and other aspects of him/her/hir self, and integrating the whole more comfortably, without overwhelm; a process demanding intuitive exercise of observation and example without prescription.

Though appreciation of strengths may sometimes play a part, this re-framing of self is not about constructing some notion of 'good person' – it is about recognizing humanity. Here Greenberg, Rice and Elliott's concepts of 'valuing and honouring the client just as he or she is now, not simply because he or she is entertaining, hard-working, or in pain' (1996, 106) and 'desiring the best for the client ... without a sense of feeling responsible for "fixing" how the client is' (1996, 107) resonate with both my commitment to respect autonomy and my concern to avoid substituting one external frame of reference with another. Clare comes to mind, persistently dominated by a ferocious inner critic, she spent the greater part of one session in particular castigating herself for having too nervous a disposition to cope with transition. Simple observations that she was 'sensitive' and 'really cared about what others may think' contributed to her re-framing perceived 'weakness' into 'consideration' – one small step on the journey to re-conceptualizing self from 'useless thing' to 'thoughtful person'. Whilst in similar circumstances the phrase 'artistic temperament' opened the door for musician Trudy to align her anxieties with her talents rather than her transsexualism, thereby holding them more comfortably and consequently experiencing noticeable reduction. Part of the process of being alongside any client is about enabling the re-framing of self and situation in order to enable movement. Simply offering my perception that what are regarded as human weaknesses can amount to strengths at too full or insufficient volume sometimes proves sufficient to facilitate clients reframing to a more comfortable and resilient way of being, as well as implicitly reminding them of their humanity.

Contrary to popular presumption I seldom find my clients confused about their gender. More often they are confounded as to how their self experienced gender might align with, and/or be accepted by those who are cisgendered. One of the ways I open discourse on gender is to lay out my own possible subjectivities as example. I have always exhibited traits and attributes common with my father, so have been aligned with him for as long as I can remember (apparently we even have the same walk, which surprisingly causes neither concern). Having respect and admiration for him, and being relatively comfortable with the gender ascribed me at birth I understand these given similarities simply as family traits. However, had I been a transsexual child such comparisons may well have had different affect. Were I female bodied but male gendered such comparisons might be constructed gender affirming – 'Of course I am like my father, I am a man too'. Conversely were I born male bodied but female gendered such constant alignment to my father might be held ridiculous, even abhorrent – 'I am nothing like my father. I am not a man!' Sometimes it is not the words themselves that hurt but how their meanings land on us. De-constructing gender stereotypes can prove a challenging and useful discussion in enabling freedom from that oppression. This is a useful exercise for therapist to think about in their training – to explore the meaning of their own body in relation to statements made by family/friends and to explore what this means, how it feels and the ways in which it has helped or hindered configuring person-hood.

Sometimes it *is* the words themselves that damage. Freud (1933, 113) noted 'When you meet a human being the first distinction you make is "male" or "female"? and you are accustomed to making the decision with unhesitating certainty'. Within the trans-identified, trans-historied, and intersex populations that certainty is frequently questioned and indeed for some may not even exist. The scene is set for controversy and conflict – because human-beings strive for fit so firmly. When we are physically and psychologically sex/gender congruent according to the binary model (cisgendered) we have the privilege of exercising any number of essentialist or constructionist arguments to validate our own experience of self; indeed we may even theorize away from those identity frameworks totally and create new ones. However if our existence itself transgresses the cisgender model then our freedoms to self define is not only interrogated by that hegemony but also distorted and often denied. Where feminist essentialism places the universality of womanhood in anatomy, transgender essentialism places this in mind/brain. Many trans' narratives concur with the observation made by Conway that it is 'probably necessary to believe in essential maleness and femaleness to have a transsexual experience' (1998, 150) and place notions of 'true gender' at the core. A stance often validated by the tragic story of David Reimer, who having been ascribed female following faulty circumcision, later transitioned back to male denouncing his clinicians' belief that gender is socially acquired. Whilst this essentialist stance proves both useful in validating surgery for those who are trans-identified and standing against surgery in the case of those born intersex; it's also a premise that subsequently colludes with binarian stereotypes, and consequently the struggles these entail. Research into Sex Difference in the Human Brain and its Relation to Transsexuality, by Zhou, Hofman, Gooren and Swaab (1995)[3] relating to the

---

3   See Zhou J.-N., Hofman M.A., Gooren L.J., Swaab D.F. (1997), *A Sex Difference in the Human Brain and its Relation to Transsexuality.* IJT 1:1 <http://www.symposion. com/ijt/ijtc0106.htm>.

opposite sexing of the BSTc in transsexual subjects further provides similar essentialist evidence for this particular population whilst subsequently colluding with the medical discourse of defect.

However, aside from academic and political circles, the mention of gender as social construct is often an anathema to transsexual and trans-historied people. Historically dubbed delusional, fabricated by mental disorder, and unreliable, the notion of any construct is too close to those moral fires for most to hold. Notions of constructing alternative identity and unsettling assumptions around sex and gender can feel extremely risky; if my client already feels out on a ledge the concept of jumping off is unlikely to feel beneficent. The concept of performativity is so conflated with the idea of pretence that very few feel able to encounter it. Learning to swim feels useful analogy here – most of us are unlikely to engage happily with this process if, when non swimmers, we are lobbed in at the deep end! There's something about engaging with the shallows, learning to play, and being able to get out, that feels important. Even when we can swim the place, style, and distance we choose to swim at will vary; similarly the context, way, and degree to which we express and explore gender. The option to swim is usually balanced with an option not to swim, and this is equally applicable to client work – else we are guilty of replacing one oppression with another – 'Go on get in! You know you like it really'. The implications of de-constructing gender can be experienced as threatening and destructive, rather than liberating, because frameworks do not simply confine us they also keep us safe. Freedom from the pressure of the frame does not necessarily comprise total removal – sometimes it's a matter of adjusting the fit.

The Nature–Nurture debate persists in the field of gender, despite growing awareness that aspects of life are multi-factorial (Ashmore 1990;[4] Spence 1999[5]). Where binarian constructs reside within the client there is something around making sure that while the client is aligning themselves with acceptability it is not collusion with oppression – without disrespecting right to autonomy. Application of anti-sectarian principles through being non-judgemental can simultaneously enable genuine respect for client autonomy whilst avoiding collusion with any oppression. Even where people find the binary comfortable, clients identifying within it but not officially accepted by it, sometimes struggle because of internalized sexism and tendency toward stereotyping. Widening the frame can be particularly challenging when the people who are oppressed parallel that very oppression, and is not without struggles. It is rare but when a client concept of femininity

    4   See Ashmore, R.D. (1990), 'Sex. Gender and the individual', in *Handbook of Personality Theory and Research*, L.A. Pervin (ed.) (New York: Guildford Press), pp. 486–526.

    5   See Spence, J.T. (1993), 'Gender-related traits and gender ideology: Evidence for a multifactorial theory', in *Journal of Personality and Social Psychology* 64 (Washington: American Psychological Association), pp. 624–635.

comprises solely notions of youthful fashion, sexual submission and/or enjoying a life of total leisure there are explorations to be made.

Being 'othered' may be endemic in all human existence. As Connolly observes 'Identity requires differences in order to be, and it converts difference into otherness in order to secure its own self-certainty' (2002, xiv). However, whilst cisgendered people may be othered through race, creed, attribute and so on, their fundamental status as people stands firm; the same is not always held true for those who are trans-identified, trans-historied, or intersex. There is something about playing the game by the rules here – it seems if one fits the rules then one can transgress them – however if one doesn't fit the rules to start with then one is simply not allowed to play the game. This may be evidenced by the pejorative radical feminist attitudes propounded by people such as Janice Raymond, whose publication *The Transsexual Empire* (1979)[6] condemned male-to-female transsexual subjectivity as the horrific result of men's womb envy; and Sheila Jeffrey's who interpreted transsexualism as internalized homophobia (1997),[7] citing realignment surgery as a form of self mutilation that should be outlawed.

Such derisive perspectives are not confined to overt gender politics but pervade culture on many fronts. McQuick epitomizes religious fundamentalist opposition saying 'God said and is still saying, "for all that do so are abomination [disgusting] unto the LORD thy God; both the transvestites and the transsexuals, all categories under transgender"; following through with the acerbic imagery "Would you put a rotten decayed dog into your house before the dining table?"' (2006, 41). Extreme opinion exists in every context – the difference between the sex and gender variant population and other marginalized groups is that the individuals concerned have precious little to counter the effect. It can for example be extremely difficult to find a lighter side of life when the lighter side frequently parodies one's existence, as in the character of Emily Howard[8] in the contemporary television series *Little Britain*.

The socialization of children to the norms of their culture is a natural process, so if a child observes no fit with that pattern, moreover perceives his/her/hir own pattern to be pilloried and persecuted, then alienation feels inevitable. Indeed

---

6   Raymond J.G. (1994) [Originally published – Boston: Beacon Press, 1979], *The Transsexual Empire: The Making of the She-male* (New York: Teachers' College Press).

7   See Jeffrey, S. (1996), 'Heterosexuality and the Desire for Gender', in *Theorising Heterosexuality: Telling it Straight*, Richardson, D. (ed.) (Buckingham: Open University Press), pp. 75–90; and (2003), *Unpacking Queer Politics: A Lesbian Feminist Perspective* (Cambridge: Polity Press).

8   'Emily Howard, played by David Walliams (real name: Eddie Howard), is an unconvincing transvestite, who dresses in Victorian dresses and insists [*sic*] that she be treated as a "lady" by always reminding people "I am a lady". He speaks using Victorian English, sprinkled with French phrases to sound more feminine. However, in certain situations, usually when he is busy, he reverts back to his normal voice or male mannerisms. Nearly everyone can recognize that he is a man, and treats him accordingly' <http://www.littlebritain.net/character-and-sketches/emily-howard.html?Itemid=27>.

research by Human Rights Watch found that 'the abuse of lesbian, gay, bisexual and transgender youth is predicated on the belief that girls and boys must strictly adhere to rigid rules of conduct, dress and appearances based on their sex'. They went on to note that: 'Regardless of their sexual orientation or gender identity, youth who violate these rules are punished by their peers and too often by adults' (Bochenek and Widney Brown 2001, 49). Cisgender sectarianism starts young, and like all sectarian beliefs is characterized by adherence to a narrow, dogmatic, viewpoint. Countering the effects of such long term negative conditions of worth entails communicating genuine acceptance of gender diversity and respect for the client's right to self governance.

Over the past decade one of the greatest frustrations reported by my trans-identified and intersex clients is antipathy toward the aspirations and expectations of their ascribed (as opposed to experienced) gender. Feeling unable to comply with these fundamental societal constructs precipitates a self concept permeated with notions of insufficiency and weakness. Consequently a major part of the therapeutic process involves affirmation of their validity as people. Similarly to Aldarondo's view of gay-affirmative therapy I believe that part of the therapists role concerns enabling the client 'to dispute, deconstruct, and subvert society's prejudicial views rather than continuing to internalize or be limited by them' (2007, 125). The key concept here being 'enabling': the introduction of some a priori political agenda, however well intended, feels well beyond the remit of most counselling, and certainly contrary to the ethical principles of autonomy and self governance in Britain. However the provision of information to enable the client to entertain wider perspectives, encounter possibilities, and make informed choice feels sometimes both appropriate and necessary.

Many trans-identified people report incidence of cross-dressing at an early age, and relate that experience to feeling relaxed, comfortable, or happy; yet extremely few will have shared this comfortable, relaxed and happy experience with their peers or family, either at the time or afterward. This is rarely because they have been told such behaviour is wrong, but because behaviours that are unspoken are quickly assumed unspeakable. Social norms so embedded in culture that knowledge of them is derived experientially, tacitly established and maintained through *body language* and *non-verbal communication* during normal social discourse, are extremely powerful. Bringing this awareness into therapeutic discourse sometimes enables clients to de-construct the oppressive frame that has been yoked on them and develop less burdensome subjectivities. Notions of trans identities and intersex bodies as sinful, abhorrent, and unnatural not only feel ubiquitous but often become internalized – to the extent that people ascribed those labels sometimes feel wholly responsible for any unhappiness, lack, and even tragedy, within both self and their immediate social group. This Jonahesque concept, compounded by societal attitudes and individuals' experience, is difficult to wrestle away. I have counselled more than one individual who accepted blame for a relative's death as resulting from the stress of their existence, as well as several who attributed absence of fertility in their marriage a result of their cross-dressing. Re-framing from perniciousness is a precarious process. Facilitating movement from blame states necessarily comprises an acute awareness of power and authority, and feels somewhat akin to the difference between educing and instruction in education. Similarly it often includes careful sharing of information, example and resources. One client's journey could be heard in the following progression over a period of years 'I am bad', 'I am a bad person', 'It's bad of me ...', 'Am I being bad?', 'I am silly aren't I?', 'That's silly of me, isn't it?', 'I did something silly but that's OK isn't it?', to a smiling 'I am a funny person', able to live more comfortably with the fallibility of being human and able to develop the necessary resilience that entails.

Kessler and McKenna (1997) note that 'the gender attribution process is an interactive one, grounded in the attributors' unshakable belief that everyone can and must be classified as female or male'. Accepting that belief and immutable fact are not synonymous is consequently often the first step in co-constructing a reframing of gender. Construction itself depends on having the tools and material from which to construct, so 'using literature for self-help and personal growth' (Kus 1995, 79) can be a valuable part of this process. All subjectivities are culturally situated, specific to and informed by the time and place in which they exist: in the future perhaps society will not need to frame gender at all – meantime for most people working away from a culturally embedded two box system is incremental, and may feel decidedly precarious. As Parsons notes 'When transsexuals try and seek out more suitable identities they can only pick from those that their society offers' (2005, 61) and until recently that has been extremely limited.

Beyond a few famous icons such as the glamorous April Ashley and erudite Jan Morris it has been virtually impossible for trans-identified people to find any positive role models to counter social slur. Expanding possible futures necessarily comprises an awareness of alternatives, and, though celebrity icons can be inspiring, most ordinary human beings cannot construe reaching such heights, especially when in distress. Moreover, whereas the cisgendered majority is raised on stories that present myriad possible futures, trans-identified and gender variant people are conspicuous by their absence in the narratives of childhood, effectively crippling their sense of place in the world from the outset. Moving from this oppression to liberty, at least initially, necessitates an understanding of options, and quite simply if people cannot see anything viable they tend to remain stuck. I have found genuine awareness of successful trans' and gender variant lives from every level of service in retail, industry, education and government, diverse in personality, attributes and political stance, helpful in facilitating this journey. Whilst Wilchins observes that 'When it comes to gender, each of us, in our own private way, is an implicit philosopher' (2002, 33) few clients feel sufficiently comfortable in themselves to contemplate, let alone attempt, gender free fall. Alternative sources of information such as the 'FtMs and female-bodied men throughout history' on YouTube <http://www.youtube.com/watch?v=ND8LVPaTZKo> and Dr Lynn Conway's 'Transsexual Women's Successes: Links and Photos' <http://ai.eecs.umich.edu/people/conway/TSsuccesses/TSsuccesses.html> have also proven helpful in enabling people to re-frame away from self prognosis of pariah to more positive possibilities.

My experience as therapist resonates with Ceri Parsons observation that the 'notion of authenticity of identity is particularly significant for transsexual people given the challenges they face in their claims to being a particular gender when their corporeality often contradicts such claims' (2005, 62). People presented with a two box system and finding the one ascribed inadequate, not only feel compelled to move, but also anxious to fit incontrovertibly in the other. The heterosexist nature of the gender binary thus adds further challenges to the construction of trans' and gender variant identity. One example of this is the way clients who experience self as female and align with other women can feel betrayed by attraction toward them. In S.V.'s case she had poured out a familiar trans-narrative of childhood cross-dressing, and an adolescence full of the angst of conflicting impulses (Did she want to be *with* her or *be* her?). The continuing paradoxes of her middle years had resulting in her becoming persistently self deprecating. Eventually she clarified her central conflict – 'It's no good! You see … I know I cannot be transsexual … I still fancy women!'

The response that fell from my mouth was 'Ever heard of lesbians?' The delivery was not flippant and whilst this response may seem closed it precipitated useful discussion about orientation, gender identity, and the possible correlations between the two thus opening new possible pathways. Being "queer squared" does not in itself provide a solution, and was not offered as such, but in this case where overwhelming focus on fit obliterated alternatives I considered it politic to expand the frame.

The hypervigilance that pervades the trans-identified population runs so high that the current DSM recognizes 'Suicide attempts and Substance-Related Disorders are commonly associated' and individuals 'may manifest coexisting Separation Anxiety Disorder, Generalized Anxiety Disorder, and symptoms of depression'. (APA 2000, 578). I would assert that this is not due to any inherent weakness in the population itself but to the damage wrought by social stigma and ostracism. Low self worth and relational anxieties neither develop nor abate in isolation; moreover they frequently mesh to reinforce each other. It seems logical that being from a marginalized minority might exacerbate fear of separation, especially from primary attachment figures. As to being anxious of scrutiny and fearful of embarrassment, these very human characteristics are inevitably magnified in a population subject to open ridicule and public scandal. Underpinning the therapeutic alliance on the client centred tenets of empathically understanding the client's subjective experience, and development of a genuine, prizing, accepting bond with the client; combined with collaboratively co-constructing more comfortable narratives can prove invaluable in negotiating safe passage through such struggles. As with any client presenting relational anxieties, it would be damagingly naïve not to engage with the possibility of loss; however it is equally credulous to assume that any diversity necessarily precipitates it. Something about facilitating perspectives and resilience feels pertinent, and these principles persist in my practice, in both explicit and implicit form.

People make sense of themselves through their stories, and perhaps more accurately, through those stories being not only heard but understood. Consequently describing a gendered experience that does not actually sit within the binary pattern presents a very awkward if not impossible task; previously explained through the analogy of 'having only black and white paint to describe a yellow brick road' (Livingstone 2008, 141). Since knowledge is situated neither client nor therapist necessarily has all the vocabulary to do this satisfactorily; consequently my work often employs imagery and analogy to widen the frame. An awareness of the diverse cultural perspectives on gender that exist in the world, such as the place of the Fafafine in Samoan society and the Native American concept of 'Two-Spirit', can also be enabling for some clients. The latter example being particularly significant for those who experience themselves as inter- or bi-gendered, as shown in the following poem:

A Daughter Yet Born A Son

In strangled words, and burning tears,
I poured out all that had for years,
Been torturing my inner state,
My Guilt, My doubt and worthless fate.

In sobbing recoil nothing kept,
As clear and honest while I wept,
In hope of answers long to find,
I laid out all my troubled mind.

In tones of affirmation might,
Like dawn to end the bleakest night,
Her wise words told without demand,
Like sea which soothes the tidal sand.

That which long I'd buried deep,
Began to surface through the sleep,
Of half life lived in anxious fear,
To understand what I hold dear.

That I am of a different kind,
Not worthless freak of deformed mind,
But of sprits two, not of one,
A daughter, yet born a son.

                                                  Veronique Jay, 2008

Beyond the binary is a diversity of experience including genderqueer, third gender, bi-gendered and agendered people – most of whom did not assign themselves in these ways simply to provide interesting examples of transgression for queer theorists! Many simply wish to have their existence given equal respect, and look to therapy for space to explore the realities of living more often than the curiousness of being. Paradoxically my experience is that whilst those presenting ordinary appearance may hold very diverse understandings of their gender those presenting as visibly queer sometimes have the most conservative narratives. Conversations with Ember, who presents very strikingly as lifestyle slave, revealed a very conservative female narrative – she explained that when she presented ordinarily she found the gape and gawp of the general public acidic, as she is now 'It is my choice they stare, not theirs'. An interesting power dynamic; and not a singular one. Another client revealed 'The piercings are a good disguise. People are so fascinated by them and the amazing hair that they do not notice me behind them'. Two clients – two ways of using apparel; there are undoubtedly a myriad more.

Where the client wishes to explore identity I believe Hodges assertion that: 'There is a very fine line between encouraging clients to question negative stereotypes and assumptions … and promoting an alignment with established identity categories' (2008, 18), is as true for gender minorities as sexual orientation. Embracing the possibilities of a rainbow doesn't necessarily involve casting out the pink and the blue. If the right to self identify beyond the binary is taken to supersede it we move dangerously close to creating alternative oppressions rather than alleviating them. Since we need words to convey our meanings, de-labelling self and society feels somewhat impractical, and besides some clients identify with current terminology and that, I feel, should be respected. What I then endeavour to do is assist the client with stripping down existing labels of regulatory discourse, co-constructing less incisive meanings, and finding alternatives where usual labels do not fit.

The following exchange shows how the premise that only male sexuality resides in erection combined with assertions that 'primary' or 'true' transsexual people are disgusted by their genitals combine as regulatory discourses bringing guilt and shame. It also illustrates how a client came to the possibility of re-framing that oppression through the sharing of information. F.N. was going through transition to female and had physically responded well to hormone therapy. Erectile dysfunction preceded clinical treatment by a year and was not considered problematic. F.N. identified as lesbian and was out on the scene, she had not yet engaged in any sexual encounters but looked forward to the possibility of intimacy sometime after surgery.

> F.N. "I think I am turning into a man!"
> [bursts into tears and reaches for tissues]
>
> T.L. "Oh my dear!"

F.N. "I am. I know I am"
[Crying continues for some minutes]

F.N. "Everything was going so well and now this. Now the hormones have gone in reverse!"

T.L. "That feels unlikely. What makes you think that?"

F.N. [tearfully] "We'd had such a wonderful day ... Such a wonderful day.
Ended up back at hers ...
Listened to music, had a chat ... had a hug ...
And then! ... God it was dreadful ... awful ... I thought I was going to die
I can't even say it

T.L. "Something unspeakable happened"

F.N. "Yes! Totally ... so bad ... so so bad ... I just left. Had to ... God knows what she thought!
[cries]

T.L. "Something stirred"

F.N. "Yes!"
[struggles to continue]
How can this happen? You know me.
I don't have those. Haven't for years.
Why me? Why now?
Do you think it's the tablets?"

T.L. "No I don't"

F.N. "Well why am I turning into a man?"

T.L. "I don't think you are"

F.N. "I must be. Either that or a monster"

T.L. "Unlikely"

F.N. "So what do you think?"

T.L. "You stopped having erections long before hormones didn't you?"

F.N. "Ages ... Yes ... It was lovely"

T.L. "And you've been depressed for some time"

F.N. "Years"

T.L. "Mmmmm ... Stress and depression can cause erectile dysfunction I believe"

F.N. "Yes I know ... But I'm a lot better now"

T.L. "Off anti-deps?"

F.N. "Yep"

T.L. "Well ... I understand that sometimes when spirits rise other things do too"

F.N. "O my God!
But what about the 'mones?"

T.L. "Not *everyone* on hormones stops having stiffies"

F.N "Really??"

T.L. "Really"

The above shows how assimilation of the classic transsexual narrative can prove truly problematic. All autobiographies are selective, as well as subjective, and when aligning ourselves to others, whatever the reason, we naturally select commonalities. However, when that narrative becomes the sole means by which we can or cannot access medical treatment it becomes even more heavily bound by regulatory discourse. A major part of classic transsexual narrative is disgust with natal genitals, vis-à-vis the sexual functions of the same, and though without doubt both are true for some people, neither is true for all. By becoming a critical part of diagnosis these stories silence other narratives and contribute to the de-humanizing of the people per se by effectively neutering their stories. Perceptions that any population's existence could rest entirely on a series of rigid immutable truths is damagingly parochial; stripping persons of their identity as possibly sexual human beings feels utterly callous. To accept that some people are asexual is totally different to the presumption that an entire population should be so – and distinguishing the two necessitates careful dialogue with the clients concerned. Some of the saddest moments in my work have occurred when having arrived at a place where partner relationships are an emotional possibility the client recounts that it is academic anyway, as having previously identified as asexual they have been persuaded to have purely cosmetic surgery.

The Second and Third Separations

Loney observes that oppressed groups 'continue to be victimized by bogus conceptions of their identity that were illegitimately imposed on them' (1998, 23). Minority groups thus tend to police their members with regulatory practices, paralleling the sectarianism that segregated them in the first place. Even if the group label fits, the individual may not wish, or indeed be able, to wear it in the same way as the others, and discourse intended to be unifying can actually re-enforce feelings of exclusion. This ironic legacy Loney notes as traceable to radical activists 'railing against the tyranny of conformity' subsequently leading to 'the development of a style of politics that imprisons its practitioners in ever-tighter confines of proliferating group identities' (1998, 42). As the group narrative becomes solidified, individuality is then silenced.

Any categorization can in this way propagate a new sectarianism. This occurs not so much through the exercise of category itself but through the subsequent notions of value, order and ranking that become implicit within it. When we create a category it becomes distinct from the other; what we then seem to lack is the ability to sustain common links. My practice feels to a great extent about re-connecting those links; re-framing sex and gender diversity so that my clients can carry it more comfortably and sustain their rightful links with the rest of humanity. When individuals are seen first and foremost as members of identity groups 'justice no longer requires treating individuals equally, but rather groups must be treated differently to accommodate the needs presumed to flow from intrinsic group characteristics' (Loney 1998, 4). Employing anti-sectarianism is about avoiding absolutism; rather than denying variety holding it safely as part of the whole.

The concept of sheltering under an umbrella may feel intrinsically beneficial but whilst sex, gender and sexuality based minorities are all prone to heterosexist persecution, they are also an inherently diverse, comprising different needs, wants and cultures. The LGB and T alliance, where it does exist, is rarely a wholly happy one by nature of its own diversity and its rather tenuous grouping. The Stonewall Riots could be taken as example of how the colonization of narrative exacerbates such divisions. These were spontaneous and violent demonstrations against a police raid that took place in the early hours of 28 June 1969 at the Stonewall Inn, Greenwich Village, New York. Frequently cited as a defining moment in history when gay and lesbian populations fought back against government-sponsored persecution, the name of Stonewall is memorialized in the title of the best known LGB association in English and American culture. Though as Riki Ann Wilchins observes 'it was drag and transpeople like Sylvia Rivera, Marsha P. Johnson, and Yvonne P. Ritter who ignited the Stonewall Rebellion' (1997, 202). The trans-identified population remain excluded in the Stonewall remit which is defined as a 'Lesbian, Gay and Bisexual Charity' except in Scotland.

More recently some have found the colonization of the life of Brandon Teena disturbing; the use of female pronouns in some writing attributing him as butch lesbian rather than transgender man.[9] And there was heated debate, protest, and counter protest, following Julie Bindel's nomination for the Stonewall 2008 Journalist of the Year Award, because of her separatist politics and previous transphobic writing. Thus, conflict within the LGB and T arena thrives on sectarian attitudes – the very thing that separated the people from the rest of the population in the first place – and disturbingly parallel.

Yet we are at the dawn of greater inclusivity, heralded with the development of groups such as Canada's young feminist Rebelles whose manifesto states:

> We are women of diverse abilities, ethnicities, origins, sexualities, identities, class backgrounds, ages and races. Among us are employed, underemployed and unemployed women, mothers, students, dropouts, artists, musicians and women in the sex trade. We state that transfolks, two-spirited and intersexed people are integral to our movement and recognize and respect gender fluidity and support the right to self-identify. Our women-only spaces include everyone who self-identifies and lives as a woman in society. <http://www.rebelles2008.org/en/manifesto>

Unfortunately we have a way to go and a few bridges to burn and build before we reach the ideological notion of true single equalities. As noted elsewhere some feminists have distinct aversions to trans-identity – so the frequently held trans to female client notion that women are more accepting does not carry the universal truth some attribute to it. Problems of misconception are not however one sided; the statement 'I'm going to the Lessie café because I know they'll be nice. After all they are manly women like me' instigated a challenging but obviously necessary re-framing discussion with one trans-historied lady in particular.

One of the major causes of unease within the trans' population concerning LGB and T alliance, is that many don't actually identify as lesbian, gay, or bisexual – they identify as heterosexual. Alignment with sexual minorities is therefore received as totally inappropriate. It is also seen to re-enforce the misconception of trans' status as sexually rather than gender based. This results in the somewhat curious paradox that while some are banging on the door to get in, others are looking for a window to climb out! One client broke down in tears when her employer drew her attention to a forthcoming LGBT meeting – she wasn't sure if it was a single slap or a double one – but as a trans-historied woman, not out as either lesbian or trans' at work, she experienced this action as hurtful rather than helpful.

Many therapists concerned with sexual minorities are keen advocates of relevant support and social groups; since where minority is marginalized due to orientation finding a group of similarly inclined people has very obvious relational advantages. However, assumptions of such community do not necessarily apply when marginalization is gender based; without sound knowledge of the actual

---

9   See Jones, A. (1996), *All She Wanted: The True Story of Brandon Teena* (New York: Pocket Books).

situation, recommending that a client attend a local support group may indeed be ill advised. The medicalization of transsexualism may have created an oasis of legitimacy for a minority with a minority but it's also exacerbated a microcosm of society itself with vehement sectarianism. James Barrett observes 'Whether transvestism is contiguous with transsexualism or distinct from it is a debate that has endured over decades' and goes on to note the 'current diagnostic position including dual-role transvestism but not fetishistic transvestism as a gender identity disorder reflects this uncertainty' (2007, 31). Uncertain or not this construct has become embedded and perpetuates sexism, stigma and sectarianism within the trans-identified population itself, as well as wider society.

Jeffrey's stance that 'men's practices of femininity are not about being 'women' but about adopting the socially prescribed behaviours of a subordinate group in order to enjoy the sexual satisfactions of masochism that this offers' (2005, 49) not only negatively sexualizes trans-identity but re-enforces the medicalized sectarianism within the trans-population itself. This confusion of sexual and gender diversity doubly increases the responsibility of the therapist to be explicitly non-judgemental, since both aspects are equally valid and fundamental parts of human life. The misconception that transsexual identity is completely gender based whilst transvestism is a totally sexual matter is not only culturally divisive it propagates problems for individuals within both diversities because of consequent pressure to conform. Clinical legitimacy may seem to provide welcome relief from the storm of stigmatization for those who meet its criteria but as it stands it perpetuates a narrative of 'wrongness'. The logic that those who do not fit the accepted gender pattern must be physically defective if not psychologically defective is profoundly heterosexist; the concept of something inherently wrong is not wrestled away, This neutering discourse does not stop with efforts to avoid fetishistic transvestism as 'being aroused by the thought of oneself as female, or with primary or secondary sexual characteristics' (Barrett 2007, 35) can now lead to diagnosis of 'autogynephilia' (Blanchard 1989). Blanchard classified autogynephilic sexual fantasies into four subtypes in 1991;[10]

- Transvestic autogynephilia: arousal to the act or fantasy of wearing women's clothing.
- Behavioral autogynephilia: arousal to the act or fantasy of doing something regarded as feminine.
- Physiologic autogynephilia: arousal to fantasies of female-specific body functions.
- Anatomic autogynephilia: arousal to the fantasy of having a woman's body, or parts of one.

---

10   See Blanchard, R. (1991), 'Clinical observations and systematic studies of autogenephilia', in *Journal of Sex and Marital Therapy* vol. 17, no. 4 (New York: Human Sciences Press), pp. 235–251.

Lest we get distracted by masturbation (a chief component of transvestic fetishism), Blanchard is quite clear that autogynephilia refers to potential for sexual excitation and that the subject does not necessarily become aroused every time – which seems to about have transsexualism taped so that asexuality is the only option. The implications for social control here are immense: since sexuality is relational many of the population duly become frozen in relationship lest it lead somewhere that negates gender identity. Perhaps it is an oversight of the patriarchy that autophallaphilia remains as yet undocumented, or maybe I simply missed the article. Anyway, those born female bodied do not seem to attract such incising discourse. The responding narrative of pre-operative asexuality remains mainly prevalent in those transitioning to female; liberating them from that regulatory discourse demanding close collaboration and genuine exploration as to whether or not this is something from which the particular client concerned needs liberating.

That some of those perceived as willingly transgressing the bounds of both sex and gender dare to engage in these transgressions on a part time basis is evidently perceived affront to heteronormative discourse. Cross-dressing remains so entrenched in stigma that the majority of people concerned find themselves castigated on all sides. Societal assumptions that transvestites are strictly motivated by sexual deviation casts them into a veritable sin pit proliferated by perceptions of wickedness, weakness, and wrongdoing; thus bringing us full circle to the concept of sex and gender diversity being morally defective. My experience is that those identifying as cross-dressers and transvestites are as diverse in personality as the rest of us; equally human, and equally subject to the stresses of being so. Perhaps reading David Walliams book *The Boy in a Dress* (2008)[11] should be compulsory curriculum not simply in counselling training but within schools.

Conclusion

Gender regulatory discourse affects us all to a degree – but seldom more keenly than when we feel our very identity ascribed inappropriately. Deconstructing and challenging normative discourses allows the development of narratives beyond the limitations of cultural oppression. More importantly, engaging with human beings as human beings enables humanity. It feels important to acknowledge that not every client seeking out specialist therapy actually wishes to enter into dialogue about their diversities. Sometimes it simply seems a more likely space to be met as a human being and engage with the issues rather than the therapist's curiosity:

I went to see the Doctor wearing make-up:

Izzard: "I've got a cough"

---

11   See David Walliams (2008), *The Boy in a Dress* (New York: HarperCollins Children's Books).

Doctor: "You've got a what?"

Izzard: "I've got a cough"

Doctor: "You're a transvestite?"

Izzard: "No. I've got a cough. I am a transvestite, but I've got a cough"

Doctor: "Well, I'd better sort the transvestite thing out. Have to refer you for that"

Izzard: "No that's not a problem. Just the cough thanks". (Izzard et al. 1998, 63)

Queering my practice comprises interrogating principles both within and beyond each particular therapeutic relationship – striving to facilitate freedom from oppressions – in collaboration with and at the pace of the client. It is about consciously interrogating the power within the therapeutic alliance, rather than denying such power exists, and enabling the re-framing of subjectivities so that they do not strangle the subject. The current system of categorizing sex and gender is not only confining it has edges that can cut most deep. My experience is that therapy can assist in easing out those edges so that healing can take place. It can also provide safe space in which clients may explore the possibilities of re-framing their own constructs or co-constructing more comfortable ones. Judith Butler notes that 'if there are no norms by which we are recognizable, then it is not possible to persist in one's own being, and we are not possible beings; we have been foreclosed from possibility' (2004, 31). My experience is that when principles of client-centredness, anti-sectarianism and queer theory are combined, client and counsellor can knock that notice of foreclosure down and pick up the possibilities of being.

References

Aldarondo, E. (2007), *Advancing Social Justice Through Clinical Practice* (New York: Routledge).

American Psychiatric Association (2000), *Diagnostic and Statistical Manual of Mental Disorders Fourth Edition Text Revision DSM-IV-TR* (Washington, DC: American Psychiatric Association).

Aragon, A.P. (2006), *Challenging Lesbian Norms: Intersex, Transgender, Intersectional, and Queer Perspectives* (New York: Harrington Park Press).

Barrett, J. (2007), *Transsexual and Other Disorders of Gender Identity: A Practical Guide to Management* (Oxford: Radcliffe Publishing).

Blanchard, R. (1991), 'Clinical observations and systematic studies of autogynephilia', in *Journal of Sex and Marital Therapy* Issue 17: 4 (New York: Routledge), pp. 235–251.

Bochenek, M. and Widney Brown, A. (2001), *Hatred in the Hallways: Violence and Discrimination Against Lesbian, Gay, Bisexual, and Transgender Students in U.S. Schools* (New York: Human Rights Watch).

Butler, J. (2004), *Undoing Gender* (New York: Routledge).

Connolly, W.E. (2002), *Identity/Difference: Democratic Negotiations of Political Paradox* (expanded edn, originally published in 1991) (Minneapolis: University of Minnesota Press).

Conway, J.K. (1998), *When Memory Speaks: Reflections on Autobiography* (New York: Knopf).

Ensler, E. (2007), *The Vagina Monologues* (New York: Villard Books).

Feinberg, L. (1998), *Trans Liberation Beyond Pink or Blue* (Boston: Beacon Press).

Freud, S. (1933), 'New introductory lectures on psycho-analysis', in *The Standard Edition of the Complete Works of Sigmund Freud*, Vol. 23 (London: Hogarth 1964).

Gamson, J. (2002), 'Must identity movements self destruct', in *Sexualities Critical Concepts in Sociology*, Plummer, K. (ed.) (London: Routledge).

Good, G. (2001), *Humanism Betrayed: Theory, Ideology and Culture in the Contemporary University* (Montreal: McGill-Queen's Press).

Greenberg, L.S., Rice, L.N. and Elliott, R. (1996), *Facilitating Emotional Change: The Moment-by-Moment Process* (New York: Guilford Press).

Heyes, C.J. (2007), *Self Transformations: Foucault, Ethics, and Normalized Bodies* (New York: Oxford University Press).

Hodges, I. (2008), 'Queer dilemmas: The problem of power in psychotherapeutic and counselling practice', in *Feeling Queer or Queer Feelings*, Moon, L. (ed.) (London and New York: Routledge).

Izzard, E., Quantick, D. and Double, S. (1998), *Eddie Izzard: Dressed to Kill* (London: Virgin Books).

Jay, T. (1999), *Why We Curse: A Neuro-Psycho-Social Theory of Speech* (Philadelphia: John Benjamins Publishing Co.).

Jeffreys, S. (2005), *Beauty and Misogyny: Harmful Cultural Practices in the West* (New York: Routledge).

Kessler, S. and McKenna, W. (1997), 'Who put the "trans" in transgender? Gender theory and everyday life', *International Journal of Transgenderism*, Special Issue, *What is Transgenderism*? <http://www.symposion.com/ijt/gilbert/kessler.htm> (accessed 20 October 2008).

Kinsman, G. (2006), 'The creation of homosexuality as a social problem', in *Moral Regulation and Governance in Canada*, Glasbeek, A. (ed.) (Toronto: Canadian Scholars Press).

Krafft-Ebing, R. von (1998 [1886]), *Psychopathia Sexualis: With Especial Reference to the Antipathic Sexual Instinct: A Medico-forensic Study*, Complete English Language Edition (New York: Arcade Publishing).

Kus, R.J. (1995), *Addiction and Recovery in Gay and Lesbian Persons* (New York: The Haworth Press).

Leary, M.R. (2001), *Interpersonal Rejection* (New York: Oxford University Press).

Livingstone, T. (2008), 'The relevance of a person-centred approach to therapy with transgendered or transsexual clients', in *Person-Centered and Experiential Psychotherapies* Issue 7: 2 (Ross-on-Wye: PCCS Books).

Loney, M. (1998), *The Pursuit of Division: Race, Gender, and Preferential Hiring in Canada* (Montreal: McGill-Queen's Press).

McIntosh, M. (2001), 'The homosexual role', in *Sexualities Critical Concepts in Sociology*, Plummer, K. (ed.) (New York: Routledge).

McQuick, O. (2006), *The Sexuality Series* (Charleston: Booksurge).

Manifesto of the Pan-Canadian Young Feminist Gathering (2008) <http://www.rebelles2008.org/en/manifesto> (accessed 23 October 2008).

Mearns, D. and Thorne, B. (2007), *Person Centred Counselling in Action*, Third Edition (London: Sage).

Morley, S. and Friend, D. (2000), *Puppetry of the Penis: The Ancient Australian Art of Genital Origami* (London: Prion).

Parsons, C. (2005), 'Exploring transsexual narratives of identity (trans)formations: A search for identity', in *The Psychology of Women Section Review* Issue 7: 2 (Leicester: British Psychological Society).

Puri, B.K. and Tyrer, P.J. (1998), *Sciences Basic to Psychiatry*, Edition 2 (Edinburgh: Churchill Livingstone).

Roberts, A. (1981), *Mental Health History Words 1913 Mental Deficiency Act* <http://www.mdx.ac.uk/WWW/STUDY/mhhglo.htm#MentalDeficiency> (accessed 2 December 2008).

Rogers, C.R. (1961), *On Becoming a Person* (Boston: Houghton Mifflin).

Rogers, C.R. (1989), 'Theory and research', in *The Carl Rogers Reader*, Kirschenbaum, H. and Henderson, V.L. (eds) (London: Constable).

Shirley (1859), 'Professional sectarianism', in *Fraser's Magazine for Town and Country* (London: John W. Parker and Son).

Weedon, C. (1999), *Feminism, Theory, and the Politics of Difference* (Oxford: Blackwell Publishing).

Wilchins, R.A. (1997), *Read My Lips: Sexual Subversion and the End of Gender* (Ithaca, NY: Firebrand Books).

Wilchins, R.A. (2002), 'Queerer bodies', in *GenderQueer: Voices from Beyond the Sexual Binary*, Nestle, J., Howell, C. and Wilchins, R.A. (eds) (Los Angeles: Alyson Books).

Zerubavel E. (2006), *The Elephant in the Room: Silence and Denial in Everyday Life* (New York: Oxford University Press).

Chapter 2

Queerying Freud: On Using Psychoanalysis with Sexual Minority Clients

Ian Hodges

The history of psychoanalytic theory[1] and practice as these relate in various ways to the experiences of sexual minority persons[2] is not only complex, multifaceted and fraught with disagreements but also evidences the deep anxieties and ambivalences that human beings experience with regard to their own and others' sexuality. This chapter is primarily concerned with the question of how we may challenge heteronormativity in psychoanalytic theory and practice. I discuss aspects of the theory and practice of psychoanalysis with reference to the individual and social construction of the experiences of persons with a minority sexual identity. I also discuss the way that queer theory enables a reconceptualization of the 'truth' of psychoanalysis, especially its relation to some of our working models of sexuality within psychotherapeutic practice. I argue that understanding the contribution of psychoanalysis (both positive and negative) ultimately takes us back to Freud, in particular that his case studies provide a starting point for considering these issues – especially those in which homosexuality figures strongly. I also discuss the ways in which analysing (discursive) power relations in psychoanalysis may offer a useful model for understanding psychoanalytic work with sexual minority clients/patients.[3]

---

1   I use the term psychoanalysis here in a broad sense to mean all 'classical' models that take Freud's canon as the key point of theoretical and practical reference.

2   Here I use the term sexual minority to refer to Lesbian, Gay, Bisexual, Intersex and Transgender persons, including those defining themselves as Queer, as this allows for inclusion of a broader range of experiences not necessarily encompassed by these particular identity terms. There are debates concerning the 'alphabet' model (LGBTIQ) for expressing the variety of categories that might fall under the term sexual identity, however here I wish to emphasize self-definition and marginalization through the use of this term 'sexual minority'.

3   Here I use the terms client/patient together to include the two most commonly used terms in psychoanalysis and psychoanalytic counselling. However I wish to fully acknowledge the different opinions on whether to use the term patient or client or something other, for example analysand. These debates concern the risks of pathologization and the implication of passivity in using the term patient, while the term client also encompasses problems, for example in relation to the construction of the relative positions of consumer and service provider and the risk of impoverishment of the complexity of the therapeutic

For many, psychoanalysis has been a site in which one was almost guaranteed to find deeply pathologizing accounts of sexual minority development and experience and thus, for many sexual minority persons, psychoanalysis figures not only as a model to be treated with suspicion but as embodying those elements of psychology/psychiatry that must be fought, resisted, challenged. I have a very powerful memory of searching for books on homosexuality in my University library as a new undergraduate in the late 1980s away from home for the first time. Of course I was searching for answers to my own struggle in coming out, both to myself and others. The one book I found was Irving Beiber et al.'s (1962) *Homosexuality: A Psychoanalytic Study.* In this text I read that I was abnormal, a product of failed development, a 'sissy-boy' who would be difficult to 'treat' and, inevitably, this was far from helpful to me with my own coming out process. Thinking back to that time in the library I remember clearly the shame and sadness I experienced in reading about these 'eminent' psychiatrists who confirmed what so much of culture was then continuing to tell lesbians, gay men and bisexuals; that we were sick and in need of a cure. I had no idea then that there were psychoanalysts who were beginning to challenge these unexamined normative beliefs. Unfortunately, anti-gay campaigners such as Joseph Nikolosi still describe this text as providing the foundation for an understanding of the pathological family dynamic that 'causes' the arrested development which ultimately leads to abnormal (homo) sexual behaviour.

There is currently renewed debate among counsellors and psychotherapists concerning attitudes among UK mental health professionals towards treatments aimed at changing sexual orientation following the publication of a study by Bartlett, Smith and King (2009). This study found that of a sample of 1,328 participants (from the BPS, UKCP, BACP and RCP)[4] who completed a questionnaire concerning their views and experiences of such treatments, 4 per cent said that they would attempt to try to change a client's orientation if they requested this, while 17 per cent said they had tried to change sexual orientation for at least one client in the past. The authors concluded that 'a significant minority of mental health professionals are attempting to help lesbian, gay and bisexual clients to become heterosexual' (p. 1).

Thus, recognizing and understanding the role of psychoanalysis and other psychotherapeutic interventions in understanding and alleviating (and at times negatively contributing to) the psychological impact of living in a still deeply heteropatriarchal culture is more important than ever. Especially given that the ever increasing complexity of routine and routinized homophobia and heteronormativity makes the oppression (especially its psychological impact) of sexual minority

---

relationship. In the first study of its kind, Ritchie, Hayes and Ames (2000) asked 147 UK adult psychiatric outpatients whether they preferred the term patient or client, 77 per cent preferred the term patient. The authors ask for greater reflection on using the term client.

4   British Psychological Society, United Kingdom Council for Psychotherapy, British Association of Counselling and Psychotherapy, Royal College of Psychiatry.

persons ever more difficult to properly comprehend and effectively challenge. However, here I want to make a case for psychoanalysis as a possible site of resistance to such oppression and to emphasize its theoretical use in providing a complex and practical understanding of the oppression of sexual minority persons, along with a model of therapeutic work which may contribute to helping sexual minority patients/clients work through the impact of growing up and making a life in a heteronormative culture.

Queer Theory, Power and Psychoanalysis

For the purposes of this chapter I begin by drawing out some key ideas and themes from queer theory. I don't offer this as a fully comprehensive account of the area but rather as my sense of what is important in queer theorizing for psychoanalytic (and other psychotherapeutic) practice. This account is also reflective of my own introduction to queer theory and practice through the work of Foucault in particular and my experiences of queer activism as a central and very concrete aspect of coming out in the early 1990s.

Queer theory offers a 'toolbox' for challenging heteronormativity through providing a complex understanding of power relations and enabling meaningful and effective resistance to them, especially in relation to gender and sexual identity. It invites a re-theorizing of psychological (and social) processes as constituted through language (discourse) but always in relation to power and authority. It provides an understanding of identity as profoundly relational, and offers a strong objection to reification along with a fundamental challenge to pathologizing discourses. Queer theory and activism took its name from the reclamation of a term of abuse – 'queer' – which was adopted by many as a new label to replace and transcend established sexual, gender and racial/ethnic categories. For queer activists, categories of gender, sexuality and race/ethnicity were not merely limiting but profoundly and dangerously (sometimes lethally) oppressive, thus queer activism was militantly anti-separatist and emphasized provocation and transgression. Queer Theory was and remains concerned with challenging heteronormativity through theoretical deconstruction, politics and activism – fundamentally it is focused upon power and resistance to power. In short, queer theory focuses upon the ways in which power gets inside our bodies, our 'hearts' and our heads (see Hodges 2008, Moon 2008 and other chapters in that collection for a fuller coverage of these issues).

The work of Michel Foucault, especially his later writing on sexuality and ethics (Foucault 1990, 1992) is arguably the most widely cited and influential in relation to queer theory and was taken up, challenged and critiqued by Judith Butler (1993, 1999) whose work continues to provide a fundamental theoretical and practical source of inspiration for queer theorists and activists. In his earlier work Foucault questioned the commonplace assumption that power acted in a repressive way, as primarily a force for denying and crushing human impulses and desires. Instead he argued that in contemporary culture power more commonly operates in a positive and productive manner. In other words, he argued that the late modern relationship between knowledge and power is productive rather than repressive. Thus, what makes Foucault's work so central to queer theory is that he offered a fully developed theory of both power and resistance and not only in relation to sexuality but also in relation to a range of other key institutions and practices, for example, the penal system, psychiatry and medicine. Thus, Foucault gave queer theory an anti-foundational framework for unravelling the taken-for-granted assumptions found in psychology and psychiatry (and other systems of knowledge), where these disciplines have authority to categorize persons and behaviours as normal or abnormal, healthy or pathological.

In this way, Foucault sidelines models of power which emphasize domination and repression and suggests that rather than saying 'no', power in contemporary Western societies is a much more positive force, tied up with knowledges that tell us who we are, how we should live, what it means to be female, male, black, white, lesbian/gay, straight and so on. Power then, operates via the often subtle and routine shaping of thought and conduct. However, these shaping forces are always open to resistance. In this way, Foucault suggested that instead of analysing power as something that *crushes* subjectivity we should undertake what he called an ascending analysis, starting form the smallest, seemingly routine everyday practices and procedures that are common place in our culture and which – in an often taken-for-granted sense – shape and mould our conduct. These practices he called 'micro-capillaries' of power and only once the detailed work of mapping these practices and techniques has been completed can we begin to link them with broader forms of regulatory regimes such as capitalism and what Foucault termed biopower or biopolitics.[5]

Thus, using this model, counselling and psychotherapy become important means through which individuals are not simply regulated through therapeutic discourse but where clients' subjectivities are shaped through moulding the ways in which clients choose to practice their freedom. In relation to psychoanalysis, Foucault (1992, Rabinow 1994) provides a key means by which to theorize the ways that psychoanalytic knowledge and practice has its effects through the production of truth concerning oneself – what Foucault termed practices of subjectification – where this term refers to the array of contemporary practices and techniques through which selves are assembled and re-assembled, shaped and re-shaped in order to produce self-regulating persons. However, these shaping forces are always open to resistance and thus queer theory also invites us to question whether psychoanalysis can be turned upon itself to be used as a site of refusal and transgression.

---

5   Foucault used the term Biopolitics to refer to the complex technical operation of power upon bodies and populations: 'By [biopolitics] I mean the endeavour, begun in the Eighteenth Century, to rationalise the problems presented to governmental practice by the phenomena characteristic of a group of living human beings constituted as a population: health, sanitation, birth-rate, longevity, race ...' (in Rabinow 1994, 73; see also Foucault, 1991).

The radical potential of psychoanalysis was identified several decades ago by feminists most notably Juliett Mitchell in her 1974 *Feminism and Psychoanalysis*. Above all, writers such as Mitchell argued that Freud's insistence that sexuality was never simply given (as heterosexual for example), but is rather moulded and constrained by external forces, which, in part, operate at an unconscious level, provided a very powerful means to argue for re-thinking our current conceptions of gender and sexual identity, especially as these relate to the oppressive structures of heteropatriarchy. Minsky (1996, xii) describes this radical potential thus:

> In stressing the central role of the unconscious in all identity (that is in everything with which we make an identification, including language and knowledge), psychoanalysis inevitably suggests that all meanings can be potentially subverted, including those of gender divisions.

Before turning to the question of sexual identity in psychoanalysis I want to clarify – from the perspective of queer theory – the ways we might understand power in psychoanalytic practice. Rose (1985, 1990, 1996) more fully explored the ways in which psychological (especially therapeutic) discourses[6] enjoin individuals to 'assemble themselves' as ethical beings, reminding us that practices of the self are always more than linguistic constructions but rather emerge from a heterogeneity of discursive and non-discursive practices, architectural forms, locales and claims to authority. So, discourse and discursive practices (for example psychoanalytic therapy) set out positions from which individuals may speak (for example, doctor and client/patient, analyst and client), they link to institutions (for example the Institute of Psychoanalysis) and they construct and enable conversations about particular objects (for example heterosexual subjects) while engendering silence concerning others (for example homosexual subjects).

Following this, Parker (1997) argues that psychoanalysis must be understood not as a search for the truth (both personal and cultural) but instead as a product of the social, political and economic forces at play which constituted the broader context of the development of Freud's ideas. He also reminds us that psychoanalytic ideas have entered into our everyday mundane psychologies, such that our very sense of self and identity are indelibly affected by Freud's writings and that this is the sense in which psychoanalysis is 'true', not as a universal description of human nature but as a key component in the cultural and social construction of selves, identities and psychologies. In this way we are in a sense produced, in part, as psychoanalytic subjects.

So from a queer perspective psychoanalytic techniques do not constitute practices for revealing the truths of human nature but are rather techniques for the construction and re-construction of selves and identities – through practices

---

6   The term discourse refers to the articulation of language with certain practices and techniques, institutional forms and relations of power. Fundamentally it refers to the relations between truth (knowledge), power and identity (self).

of subjectification. Thus, I am arguing here that applying queer theory to therapy invites us to understand therapeutic practices and techniques as key elements in the contemporary exercise of government and authority (Hodges 2002, 2003, 2008). As Miller and Rose (1994, 59) have argued, the rise of therapeutics is closely tied to the rise of advanced liberalism as a 'mode of government' because it has made possible the government of conduct through the shaping of the ways in which individuals practice their freedom and for which they require guidance from experts of the 'soul' (for example psychoanalysts).

A Foucaultian framework then, offers a means of reflecting upon the 'psy' sciences through a developed theory of the operation of power in relation to language and through which we might understand the regulatory nature (power) of psychoanalytic discourse. Furthermore, Foucault's later work on sexuality – with its emphasis upon self-regulation and self-discipline – enables a consideration of the therapeutic transformation of selves as a form of subjectification (involving truth-telling) in which the ethical operation of psychotherapeutic discourse offers a way of understanding how the discourse (and concomitantly, power) gets 'inside' the subject (here the client/patient). It is not that therapy and counselling (including radical techniques) are somehow wrong or even oppressive (though this cannot be ruled out) but rather that we need to properly understand their operation both upon individuals and within society before we can make any proper evaluation. Foucault had surprisingly little to say about psychoanalysis and did not offer any developed arguments concerning it, however he does address psychoanalysis in various parts of his work, (for example, Foucault 1980, 1990, 2001). In fact it has been argued that Freud inhabits much of Foucault's writing as an unstated presence (Hutton 1988).

For Foucault, the Enlightenment was less about liberation but rather a period of ever increasing means of disciplining behaviour. For him there is no such thing as human nature, it is not something to be discovered through psychoanalysis but rather a *product* of the techniques and forms of enquiry we have invented to probe its secrets. While Foucault's early work on asylums (Foucault 2001) asked us to consider the ways that external forces (for example the power and authority of psychiatry/medicine) produced (regulated) the contours of the mind and constituted 'dividing practices' (dividing persons/bodies into 'sane' or 'mad' for example), his later work on sexuality moved towards an analysis of how persons (minds and bodies) become self-regulating. In this vein, as I have already suggested, for Foucault psychoanalysis is not a means to uncover a truth waiting to be discovered (whether based in biology, psychic apparatuses or processes and so on) but rather a range of techniques for the *construction* of the truth of the psyche:

> Our conception of the psyche, Foucault contends, has been sculpted by the techniques that we have devised to probe its secrets, to oblige it to give up hidden knowledge that will reveal to us the truth about who we are. Psychoanalysis is from a historical perspective a late addition to that enterprise, born of a long but erratic lineage of techniques for the care of the self. (Hutton 1988, 121)

Thus, for Foucault the ultimate aim of psychoanalysis is to produce self-management and self-regulation in clients/patients and comes at the end of a long genealogy of techniques for regulating self and sexuality. Hutton (1988, 131) goes on to argue that if for Freud it is understanding our sexuality that empowers our selves, for Foucault it is our will to gain power over our sexuality (after Nietzsche) that produces our desire for self-knowledge. Moreover, for Foucault the act of interpretation discovered by Freud (along with those discovered by Marx and Nietzsche), can never lead to an underlying truth, rather instead psychoanalytic interpretation moves the chain of signification along to other points in the chain and therefore may be considered a violent, possibly traumatic technique:

> There is nothing absolutely primary to interpret, for after all everything is already interpretation, each sign is in itself not the thing that offers itself to interpretation but an interpretation of other signs … Indeed, interpretation does not clarify a matter to be interpreted, which offers itself passively; it can only seize, and violently, an already-present interpretation, which it must overthrow, upset, shatter with the blows of a hammer. (Foucault 1994, 275)

Queer theory then, gives us the tools required to prize open the workings of psychoanalysis both as theory and analytic technique in such a way as to question its claims to (the discovery of) truth and to unravel its unexamined heteronormative assumptions, while at the same time allowing us to think through the ways in which psychoanalysis may offer a site of resistance to sexual prejudice and oppression via theories of the role of the (social) unconscious in the formation of identity. Queer theory tells us that the identity categories we routinely use such as lesbian/gay or straight are social and cultural products which bear the traces of culture, power, politics and history *within* them. Thus identity categories are tied up with complex chains of signification and draw powerful associations which can be very harmful, for example between homosexuality and abnormality. This is more than a concern over reification but rather an analysis of the complex forms that reification may take and the ways these work in the service of power.

Queerying Psychoanalysis in Working with Sexual Minority Clients/Client/Patients

Having outlined an argument for a queer re-reading of classical psychoanalysis as providing a radical departure from its presentation as a theory of universal human nature, in this section I now discuss the complex and often ambivalent relation between psychoanalysis and minority sexual identity and begin to think through what queerying Freud might mean for the practice of psychoanalysis with sexual minority patients/clients. I have argued that queer theory asks us to recognize the social, political and moral forces that shaped and continue to shape psychoanalytic theory and practice, especially as these relate to sexual identity and that Foucault's ideas concerning power and knowledge enable a radical rethinking of the 'truth' of psychoanalytic theory and practice. As Butler (2002, 226) has described, a key theme in Foucault's thought is an enduring 'disobedience to the principles by which one is formed' and queer theory also enables us to understand psychoanalysis (separated from its foundation in heteronormative assumptions) as providing a potential site of resistance to heteropatriarchy, especially through the way that an account of the role of the unconscious in the formation of identity allows us to model a continuity between psyche and society/culture, inside and outside. Freud's position (within his writings) on homosexuality was complex and contradictory and this probably reflected his own feelings about sexuality along with the prevailing constructions of homosexuality at the time he was working. An example of this mixture of 'liberal' (for the time) yet somewhat ambivalent positions especially with regard to aetiology and 'cure', can be found in Freud's often quoted statement on homosexuality found in his 1935 letter to an American mother who had written to him stating her concerns about her son's homosexuality (transcribed below):

Dear Mrs …

I gather from your letter that your son is a homosexual. I am most impressed by the fact that you do not mention this term yourself in your information about him. May I question you, why you avoid it? Homosexuality is assuredly no advantage, but it is nothing to be ashamed of, no vice, no degradation, it cannot be classified as an illness; we consider it to be a variation of the sexual function produced by a certain arrest of sexual development. Many highly respectable individuals of ancient and modern times have been homosexuals, several of the greatest men among them (Plato, Michelangelo, Leonardo Da Vinci, etc.). It is a great injustice to persecute homosexuality as a crime, and cruelty too. If you do not believe me, read the books of Havelock Ellis.

By asking me if I can help, you mean, I suppose, if I can abolish homosexuality and make normal heterosexuality take its place. The answer is, in a general way, we cannot promise to achieve it. In a certain number of cases we succeed in developing the blighted germs of heterosexual tendencies which are present in every homosexual, in the majority of cases it is no more possible. It is a question of the quality and the age of the individual. The result of treatment cannot be predicted.

What analysis can do for your son runs in a different line. If he is unhappy, neurotic, torn by conflicts, inhibited in his social life, analysis may bring him harmony, peace of mind, full efficiency whether he remains a homosexual or gets changed. If you make up your mind he should have analysis with me – I don't expect you will – he had [sic] to come over to Vienna. I have no intention of leaving here. However, don't neglect to give me your answer.

Sincerely yours with kind wishes,

Freud

P.S. I did not find it difficult to read your handwriting. Hope you will not find my writing and my English a harder task.

This letter provides such a useful example because we can see at once a liberal position (especially for 1935), '… it is nothing to be ashamed of, no vice, no degradation, it cannot be classified as an illness', combined with a reference to the possibility of a 'cure', '… in a certain number of cases we succeed in developing the blighted germs of heterosexual tendencies which are present in every homosexual …', along with the notion of a somehow failed development. However, Freud then suggests that analysis would help the son gain 'peace of mind' but then reintroduces the possibility of 'cure' with the clause 'whether he remains a homosexual or gets changed'. Such ambivalence runs throughout psychoanalysis. It has been argued that Freud's conflicting, sometimes 'radical', sometimes pathologizing, statements and theories concerning homosexuality ultimately led to opposing positions on homosexuality within the profession as it stands today (for example Lewes 1989, May 1995, Izzard 1999).

Freud's cases (for example 1905, 1909) have exerted a tremendous influence both as psychoanalytic documents and as works of literature and it is here that we can find more evidence of the complex and sometimes contradictory representation of homosexuality in psychoanalytic thought. Within Freud's complete psychological works Storr (2001) identified 133 cases mentioned in passing, with six properly developed accounts of individual patients. Of those six, two patients were not directly analysed by Freud: 'Judge Shreber', this case study was based on his memoirs, and 'Little Hans' where the child's father acted as an intermediary. This leaves four cases which were actually analysed directly by Freud: 'Dora', the 'Female homosexual', the 'Wolf-man' and the 'Rat-man'. Of these four cases homosexual impulses play a major role in three. Much has been written about these case studies and here I wish only to highlight the theme of homosexuality which runs through them. Moreover, it has been argued that these studies show, in fact, how homosexuality is 'structurally situated in the inaugural moments of psychoanalysis' (Fuss 2004, 45).

Dora (Ida Bauer 1882–1945) was treated for 11 weeks in 1900 and Freud entitled her case study a 'fragment of an analysis of a case of hysteria'. Dora was 18 years old, a daughter of an unhappily married couple and had a 'crush' on Frau K (a married friend of her parents), Herr K had made sexual advances to Dora when she was 15. Freud's interpretation was that Dora's crush was a screen for her unconscious and unacknowledged desire for Herr K. The unnamed 'female homosexual' whose case was entitled 'the psychogenesis of a case of homosexuality in a woman' referred to a patient who was also 18 years old and Freud discontinued treatment with her after a brief period. Freud suggested she was not ill, in fact it was her parents who had brought her to therapy following a suicide attempt. Just prior to this the patient's father had observed his daughter with her female lover. Freud described the patient as manifesting a negative transference based on a hatred of her father and of men in general. He ended the treatment early and recommended that she sought help from a female doctor.

The 'Rat-man' (thought to be Ernst Lancer, 1878–1914) was treated for 11 months from October 1907 onwards. Freud gave this study the subtitle 'From the history of an infantile neurosis'. Lancer was a 29-year-old lawyer who was experiencing obsessional thoughts, including fears that something awful would happen to people he knew, especially his father (despite the fact that his father had died several years earlier). His worst obsession concerned a punishment he heard about while in the army, which consisted of tying a pot containing rats to the posterior of an offender such that they would gnaw into the man through the anus. Freud suggested that these obsessional thoughts disguised unacknowledged homosexual phantasies and claimed to have succeeded in removing the patient's obsessions, though there was no long term follow-up from Freud who wrote that the patient was killed during the First World War.

Thus, Homosexuality and ambivalence towards it (via a mixture of liberal and pathologizing accounts) is a complex theme which runs through several of Freud's best known case studies. Indeed Fuss (2004) makes a convincing argument for the *centrality* of homosexual impulses in Freud's case studies. Fuss asks 'where is female homosexuality to be found in psychoanalysis?' and suggests that, in fact, it forms the very foundations of psychoanalytic theory. For Fuss (2004, 44) both Freud and later theorists, for example Kristeva and Lacan, all place pre-Oedipality (that is a certain arrest of sexual development) as central to the nature of the homosexual subject:

> From Sigmund Freud to Julia Kristeva, pre-oedipality defines the fundamental psychic organisation of the homosexual subject who never, it seems, fully accedes to the position of subject but who remains in the ambiguous space of the precultural ... what we see in psychoanalysis' positioning and repositioning of homosexuality is a critical fall back to the earliest stages of the subject's formation.

For Fuss, it is 'the fall', a return, a regression, that continues to define the homosexual subject in psychoanalysis and of course this trope brings with it a rich range of associations, cultural and literary, including a return to an earlier developmental phase, a lack of maturity and the 'fallen woman'. From a queer perspective we might wonder to what extent the figure of the homosexual in these cases serves to set the boundaries for a taken-for-granted, 'normal' heterosexual identity, centred around the act of procreation (cf. Domenici 1995). Thus the key model here is a 'fall' into primary identification, that is back to a pre-Oedipal bond with the mother, which in turn reflects Freud's (and the wider culture's) heteronormative assumptions and has ultimately contributed to the continued construction of homosexuality as 'other'. Moreover, we see here, with the notion of a return to pre-Oedipality, the construction within psychoanalysis of sexuality as fundamentally tied to the relations between identification and desire, and most importantly the development of these relations is primarily theorized in terms of the Oedipus complex[7] which is presented by Freud as a fundamental model of the basis for the constitution of gendered subjectivity and identity. Indeed, Lewes (1989, 64–65) suggests that all four of Freud's main aetiological models of homosexuality revolve around the Oedipus complex:

> Many of the arguments about the 'unnaturalness' of homosexuality maintain that the persistence of homosexual object choice is prima facie evidence either that the Oedipus complex has not been worked through or that its experience was so traumatic that it caused a major psychosexual regression to a primitive pre-oedipal stage.

Thus, psychoanalytic theories of the homosexual subject centre around the notion of an inverted or 'negative' resolution of the Oedipus complex.

Taking a queer position towards psychoanalysis enables us to ask that if we agree that our sexual (libidinal) energies are initially 'polymorphous', such that culture and society, socialization and family dynamics have to channel them into a heterosexual matrix, where does queer theory leave practitioners with respect to the 'truth' of the Oedipus complex? In other words, how can the radical potential of psychoanalysis be harnessed in working with sexual minority patients/clients? How can the notion of desire as produced by the forcing of libido through a matrix of signification (cf. Fink 1997, Dean 2004), as opposed to originating in biological/ anatomical forms, be used not only to understand the nature of heteronormative oppression but to challenge it in the clinical setting? These are complex questions and here I want to address one aspect of these issues; what it means if we reject the universalizing truth claims in classical psychoanalysis (and to a lesser extent the Lacanian formulation of the paternal function), and consider instead the use of the myth of Oedipus rather as a reflection and description of dominant power relations.

---

7   The Oedipus complex is commonly defined as 'a desire for sexual involvement with the parent of the opposite sex and a concomitant sense of rivalry with the parent of the same sex' (*Encyclopedia Britannia*). In Freud's own words 1900, 262): '... it is the fate of all of us, perhaps, to direct our first sexual impulse towards our mother and our first hatred and our first murderous wish against our father. Our dreams convince us that this is so. King Oedipus, who slew his father Laïus and married his mother Jocasta, merely shows us the fulfillment of our own childhood wishes'. Put another way, the 'Oedipus complex' refers to repressed wishes, desires and emotions focused around the child's relationship (usually seen as involving rivalry and castration fears in boys) with its parents.

The culture bound and heterocentric nature of Freud's notion of Oedipus has been identified by several commentators, most notably Fromm (1982, 61):[8]

> Freud considered the bourgeois family as the prototype of all families and ignored the very different forms of family structure and even the complete absence of the "family" in other cultures ... Had Freud thought of the family life among the poorer classes of his time, where children lived in the same room with their parents and were witnesses to their intercourse routinely, this early experience [the primal scene] would not have seemed so important ...

This observation returns us, once again, to the theme of the unexamined heteronormative assumptions in psychoanalysis (remember though that psychoanalysis is far from the only therapeutic model to contain such assumptions). How can queer theory help us to understand these normative models of gender and sexuality as they operate in psychoanalytic theories of sexual development and how is it possible to challenge them? I very much concur with Izzard (2000) who argues that first and foremost psychoanalysis offers a rich and complex understanding of human beings while emphasizing the value of psychoanalysis in understanding the psychological effects of oppression (2000, 112):

> I believe a major contribution of the psychoanalytic approach to be the emphasis on shame and self-hatred which is the gay, lesbian or bisexual person's inheritance of growing up in a homophobic world ... A widely regarded strength of the analytic approach is the emphasis on the experience of early life.

Psychoanalysis also helps us to recognize and understand those (often irrational) aspects of our selves that we find difficult to even acknowledge, as Budd and Rusbridger (2001, 2) argue:

> ... we [psychoanalysts] deal with the unknown and the irrational, the left out, the bits that do not add up and, above all, the parts of ourselves that we have lost because we don't want to know about them.

Here, I also wish to argue for the importance of understanding the transmission of (oppressive) values across generations as something that a) we must more fully address if we are to properly comprehend the effects of homophobia; and b) as a key means of understanding and working with the nature and operation of this transmission with clients/patients. Eve Sedgewick, in her (2004) chapter entitled 'How to bring your kids up gay', argues that so-called revisionist psychoanalysis still retains a deeply oppressive understanding of gay youth and this understanding, she suggests, is haunted by the abject 'effeminate boys', though this observation is also relevant

---

8   See also Suzanne Izzard's very useful chapter in Davies and Neal (2000) for an overview of key critiques of classical psychoanalysis as it relates to LGB clients.

to the notion of 'masculine girls'. She reviews the revisionist psychoanalytic work of Freedman (1988) and convincingly argues that such work is fundamentally a tissue of lies aimed to:

> ... convince parents that their hatred and rage at their effeminate sons really is only a desire to protect them from peer-group cruelty – even when the parents name *their own* feelings as hatred and rage. (Sedgewick 2004, 77, original emphasis)

To what extent does this parental fear, anxiety or even hatred of gender 'reversal' in their children remain the abject of current (more liberal) psychoanalytic versions of sexual orientation? This brings us back to Freud's 1935 letter considered earlier. There is no mention of the mother suggesting that her son is in distress (although of course he may have been) but rather it is the mother's distress which Freud seems to reflect in his letter. However, despite these problems, can an understanding of Oedipal relations still be helpful in working with sexual minority clients/patients? I suggest that the broad model of Oedipal relations and the complexes of desires and emotions to which it refers may not only help to make sense of the formation of gendered and sexual subjectivity through an understanding of power relations and normalization as they operate both within and without the family but may also help us to identify and understand the nature and role of the desires of parents, especially with respect to their own fears and anxieties about gender and sexuality. In other words, these ideas can help us to make sense of broader constructions of family and sexuality now in our contemporary present.

In her influential text *Bodies that Matter*, Butler (1993) aims to address the, until then neglected, role of the body in theories of discourse. She tackles the problem of the focus on the discursive construction of identities which, while offering a useful theory of power, tells us very little about structures of subjectivity and especially motivation (for example, why would an individual take up one particular discourse as opposed to another) and she argues that we require non-essentialist theories of embodiment which can account for its discursive (performative) construction. For Butler, this performative construction of the body operates as much through exclusion as through repetition:

> The normative force of performativity – its power to establish what qualifies as "being" – works not only through reiteration, but through exclusion as well. And in the case of bodies, those exclusions haunt signification as its abject borders or as that which is strictly foreclosed: the unliveable, the nonnarrativizable, the traumatic. (Butler 1993, 188)

The notion of the 'abject' signifies something or (someone) that is outside of the symbolic, sometimes violently cast out. Often the example of a corpse is given, here the abject causes repulsion as we recognize the corpse as human but it is no longer a part of the world, it should be human/alive but it isn't, (this links to Freud's notion of the uncanny). Thus the notion of the 'abject' – or a space of abjection – taken from Kristeva, as something in between object and subject, is useful here in thinking about the ways in which the lesbian/gay body through socialization and 'development' is routinely taught to doubt and question or even to hate itself. This links to notions of the 'other' and 'othering' and we might draw on the ideas of Derrida here to understand the profoundly ideological content of identity categories especially in their operation as binary systems. How then can we use psychoanalysis to bring forth and acknowledge the abject, the outcast, unspoken elements of sexual identity without (re-)pathologizing them? (How) can a revised model of oedipal relations contribute to the operation of psychoanalysis apart from its ingrained heteronormative assumptions? Drescher (2001, 121) reminds us that psychoanalytic theories play a pivotal role in practice not least because they affect our clinical skills, especially the ways we listen to and hear what clients/patients are saying, 'Because analytic theories inevitably affect therapeutic listening, the impact of a therapist's etiological theory in doing clinical work with gay men cannot be underestimated'.

Hacking (1995, 21) suggests that descriptions (discourses) of certain kinds of person generate expectations from those in authority – those experts able to offer the description – and operate within a feedback loop consisting of the constitutive elements of expert descriptions and the need for these descriptions to respond to changes in patterns of behaviour which they subsequently are unable to capture. Hacking terms this process 'the looping effect of human kinds':

> People classified in a certain way tend to conform to or grow into the ways that they are described; but they also evolve in their own ways, so that the classifications and descriptions have to be constantly revised.

This 'looping effect' refers to more than the linguistic construction of reality but suggests that sense of self is intricately bound up with the production of knowledges concerning it. With regard to psychoanalytic practice, we might usefully attend to Hacking's (op cit. 68) suggestion that:

> ... constructed knowledge loops in upon people's moral lives, changes their sense of self-worth, re-organizes and re-evaluates the soul.

Following this, I argue that taking a queer position on the 'truth' of psychoanalysis (that is, recognizing instead its status as a fiction which functions in truth), while eschewing a naïve realism equally does not then entail a naïve relativism. Rather we must acknowledge the materiality of the effects of knowledge (discourse) and its interaction with the extra discursive. As Kirk and Miller (1986, 11) suggest 'reality does not tolerate all understandings of it equally'. In this way, psychoanalytic discourse can be understood as offering clients/patients new ways of understanding themselves; new ways of describing their histories, their present experiences and their future goals. These descriptions – often offered within psychoanalytic practice as objective and factual – provide clients/patients with the possibility of changing their idea of the person they take themselves to be. Thus, psychoanalysis (including conceptions of Oedipal relations) can be considered as a discursive practice which not only (re-)constructs conduct (for example through our sometimes lost narratives of how our past has led to our present) in an ethical way, (that is, in such a way at to affect our sense of worth, our multiple moral locations), but also as a practice which responds to changes in behaviour via the interpretation of discourses and narratives we use in therapy to account for the kinds of human beings we take our selves to be. In other words, we must understand psychoanalytic practices as, in part, co-constructions but where power (both within and without the consulting room, these cannot be separated) figures centrally. It is crucial therefore that the complexes and forms of relations represented by the myth of Oedipus be understood as both a product and to some extent a description, of the social/cultural (heteronormative) forces which govern and shape our individual, familial and collective conduct.

Where then do these theories and arguments, which refute the (absolute) 'truth' of Freudian theory, leave us in understanding power, sexual identity and gender with respect to psychoanalytic work with sexual minority clients/patients? Rather than conceptualizing the Oedipus complex as a description of the 'natural' unfolding of childhood identification and desire within families which, by definition, will eventually lead to the formation of heterosexual subjectivity and where any other outcome signals an arrest of 'normal' development, Oedipus can be understood from a queer perspective in two different ways. Firstly, as a description of what society and culture, working through the desires of parents and care-givers, *demands* of families and children; that ultimately they produce heterosexual adults. Secondly, as pointing to the complexity of the ways in which families regulate (consciously and unconsciously) the (gendered) behaviour of children through socializing them into a mutually exclusive relationship between identification and desire, (such that identification must be same-sex and desire must be opposite sex).

That such demands do not always 'work' testifies to the polymorphous nature of desires and the multiplicity of outcomes in terms of same/other sex identification and desire. In fact, Lewes (1989) has argued (in an almost mathematical way) that there are several possible outcomes to the Oedipus complex, however while this usefully moves us on from the oppressive, normalizing force of the classical model, I argue that queer theory allows for a much more fluid and dynamic conceptualization of identification and desire where emphasis should be placed on the concrete workings and operations of power (through familial and other socialization) in the shaping and production of gender and sexual identity rather than some notion of a final outcome.

One way forward is to identify the links between the aims of queer theory and what we do in the clinical setting, Watson (2004, 74) suggests some similarities between queer theory and analytic practice thus:

Being "queer", then, is perhaps to be like someone in therapy; that is, to be a person in flux, contesting boundaries, eliding definition and exhibiting the constructedness of categorization. It is a process of problematizing and scrutinizing the genealogy of categories and throws into focus the inadequacies of binary distinctions as referents of experience (but which also enable and constrain).

However, such a 'being queer' involves much more than the scrutinizing of gender, sexual and other categories by/for the client/patient, it involves scrutinizing our own assumptions and categorizations as psychoanalysts and counsellors (and human beings) and a wider scrutiny and continual challenging of the (heteronormative) categories and assumptions within (and without) psychoanalysis itself.

Conclusion

Here I have argued for a more complex understanding of the 'truth' of psychoanalysis. From a queer theory perspective all knowledge is articulated with power and evidences the various traces of its historical development; psychoanalysis as a system of knowledge is no exception. Queer theory leaves us with the question of whether psychoanalysis can be used – with a reworking of Oedipus as a culturally constructed account of dominant Western bourgeois family (power) relations and values – to understand heteronormativity and heteropatriarchy in culture and its impact on individuals. Addressing this question would necessarily require that psychoanalysis is turned against itself, used as a tool to dismantle the heterosexist, homophobic aspects of its own models and practices.

I have presented a queer questioning of the truth of psychoanalysis, but at the same time have acknowledged its 'truth effects' and the ways it tells us something about the heteronormative assumptions within our culture (along with psychoanalytic discourse itself) which have shaped the psychic structures of sexual minority (and other) persons in sometimes oppressive and damaging ways. Such a queer reworking of psychoanalysis allows us to recognize and understand the origins and consequences of the damage done by a culture which teaches the queer body to question and sometimes even to hate itself without re-pathologizing sexual minority experience and lifestyles.

The theory and practice of psychoanalysis offers a complex and rich understanding of heteronormativity as it operates within culture and within and upon individuals. The notion of Oedipus (removed from its underpinnings in anatomy and the primacy of genital reproduction), can be turned around, twisted, (as with the notion of queer) to help us understand the way that familial and other socialization (and therapeutic, especially psychoanalytic discourse), routinely operates to silence homosexual subjectivity, producing it as abject. The complex of fears, desires and rivalries that Freud described using the myth of Oedipus can be used to diagnose the ways that dominant western family dynamics, especially the ways these produce gendered positions for children, powerfully contribute to the inter-generational transmission of abjection and the pathologizing of queer experience in such a way that produces a profound reproduction of heteronormativity. Thus, a queer reading of psychoanalysis invites us to use it against such reproduction in the service of challenging and questioning the complex and formative ways that gendered subjectivity is produced, allowing us to contribute to the construction of sexual minority identity and experience as healthy and normal through dismantling heteronormativity rather than through a search for the 'causes' of sexual minority desire.

References

Bartlett, A., Smith, G. and King, M. (2009), 'The response of mental health professionals to clients seeking help to change or redirect same-sex sexual orientation', *BMC Psychiatry* 9, 11.

Bieber, I. (1962), *Homosexuality: A Psychoanalytic Study* (New York: Basic Books).

Budd, S. and Rusbridger, R. (2005), *Introducing Psychoanalysis* (London: Routledge).

Burchell, G., Gordon, C. and Miller, P. (eds) (1991), *The Foucault Effect: Studies in Governmentality* (Hemel Hempstead: Harvester Wheatsheaf).

Butler, J. (1993), *Bodies that Matter: On the Discursive Limits of Sex* (London: Routledge).

Butler, J. (1999), *Gender Trouble: Feminism and the Subversion of Identity* (London: Routledge).

Butler, J. (2002), 'What is critique? An essay on Foucault's virtue', in Ingram (ed.).

Davies, D. and Neal, C. (2000), *Therapeutic Perspectives on Working with Lesbian, Gay and Bisexual Clients* (Maidenhead: Open University Press).

Dean, T. (2004), 'Lacan and queer theory', in Rabaté (ed.).

Domenici, T. (1995), 'Exploding the myth of sexual psychopathology: A deconstruction of Fairburn's anti-homosexual theory', in Domenici and Lesser (eds).

Domenici, T. and Lesser, R. (eds) (1995), *Disorienting Sexuality: Psychoanalytic Reappraisals of Sexual Identities* (London: Routledge).

Drescher, J. (2001), *Psychoanalytic Therapy and the Gay Man* (New Jersey: Analytic Press).

Faubion, J. (ed.) (1998), *Essential Works of Michel Foucault, Volume II: Aesthetics, Method and Epistemology* (London: Allen Lane).

Fink, B. (1999), *A Clinical Introduction to Lacanian Psychoanalysis: Theory and Technique* (Cambridge, MA: Harvard University Press).

Foucault, M. (1980), 'The confession of the flesh', in Gordon (ed.).

Foucault, M. (1990), *The History of Sexuality Volume One: An Introduction* (London: Penguin).

Foucault, M. (1991), 'Governmentality', in Burchell et al. (eds).

Foucault, M. (1992), *The Use of Pleasure: The History of Sexuality Volume Two* (London: Penguin).

Foucault, M. (1994), 'Nietzsche, Freud, Marx', in Faubion (ed.).

Foucault, M. (2001), *Madness and Civilization* (London: Routledge).

Freeman, R. (1988), *Male Homosexuality: A Contemporary Psychoanalytic Perspective* (New Haven: Yale University Press).

Freud, S. (1900/1991), *The Interpretation of Dreams* (London: Penguin).

Freud, S. (1905/1980), *Case Histories I: 'Dora' and 'Little Hans'*, Pelican Freud Library, Vol. 8 (London: Penguin).

Freud, S. (1909/1984), *Case Histories II: 'Rat Man', Schreber, 'Wolf Man', Female Homosexuality*, Pelican Freud Library, Vol. 9 (London: Penguin).

Freud, S. (1951), 'Letter to an American Mother', *American Journal of Psychiatry* 107, 787.

Fromm, E. (1982), *Greatness and Limitations of Freud's Thought* (London: Abacus).

Fuss, D. (2004), 'Freud's fallen women', in Warner (ed.).

Gordon, C. (ed.) (1980), *Power/Knowledge: Selected Interviews and Other Writings 1972–1977 by Michel Foucault* (Hemel Hempstead: Harvester Wheatsheaf).

Hacking, I. (1995), *Rewriting the Soul: Multiple Personality and the Sciences of Memory* (Princeton, NJ: Princeton University Press).

Hodges, I. (2002), 'Moving beyond words: Therapeutic discourse and ethical problematisation', *Discourse Studies* 4(4), 455–479.

Hodges I. (2003), 'Broadcasting the audience: Radio therapeutic discourse and its implied listeners', *International Journal of Critical Psychology* 7, 74–101.

Hodges, I. (2008), 'Queer dilemmas: The problem of power in psychotherapeutic and counselling practice', in Moon (ed.).

Hutton, P. (1988), 'Foucault, Freud and the technologies of the self', in Martin et al. (eds).

Ingram, D. (ed.) (2002), *The Political* (London: Blackwell).

Izzard, S. (1999), 'Oedipus – baby or bathwater? A review of psychoanalytic theories of homosexual development', *British Journal of Psychotherapy* 16(1), 43–55.

Izzard, S. (2000), 'Psychoanalytic psychotherapy', in Davies and Neal (eds).

Kirk, J. and Miller, M. (1986), *Reliability and Validity in Qualitative Research*, Qualitative Research Methods Series, Vol. 1 (Newbury Park, CA: Sage).

Lewes, K. (1989), *The Psychoanalytic Theory of Male Homosexuality* (New York: Meridian).

Martin, L., Gutman, H. and Hutton, P. (eds) (1988), *Technologies of the Self: A Seminar with Michel Foucault* (London: Tavistock).

May, R. (1995), 'Re-reading Freud on homosexuality', in Domenici and Lesser (eds).

Miller, P. and Rose, N. (1994), 'On therapeutic authority: Psychoanalytical expertise under advanced liberalism', *History of Human Sciences* 7(3), 29–64.

Minsky, R. (1996), *Psychoanalysis and Gender* (London: Routledge).

Mitchell, J. (1974), *Psychoanalysis and Feminism* (London: Allen Lane).

Moon, L. (2008), *Feeling Queer or Queer Feelings? Radical Approaches to Counselling Sex, Sexualities and Genders* (London: Routledge).

Moon, L. (2008), 'Queer(y)ing the heterosexualisation of emotion', in Moon (ed.).

Parker, I. (1997), *Psychoanalytic Culture: Psychoanalytic Discourse in Western Society* (London: Sage).

Rabaté, J. (ed.) (2004), *The Cambridge Companion to Lacan* (Cambridge: Cambridge University Press).

Rabinow, P. (1994), *Ethics: The Essential Works of Foucault 1954–1984, Vol. 1* (London: Penguin Press).

Ritchie, C., Hayes, D. and Ames, D. (2000), 'Patient or client? The opinions of people attending a psychiatric clinic', *Psychiatric Bulletin* 24, 447–450.

Rose, N. (1985), *The Psychological Complex: Psychology, Politics and Society in England 1869–1939* (London: Routledge & Kegan Paul).

Rose, N. (1990), *Governing The Soul: The Shaping of The Private Self* (London: Routledge).

Rose, N. (1996), *Inventing Our Selves: Psychology, Power and Personhood* (Cambridge: Cambridge University Press).

Sedgewick, E. (2004), 'How to bring your kids up gay', in Warner (ed.).

Storr, A. (2001), *Freud: A Very Brief Introduction* (Oxford: Oxford University Press).

Warner, M. (ed.) (2004), *Fear of a Queer Planet: Queer Politics and Social Theory* (Minneapolis: University of Minnesota Press).

Watson, K. (2005), 'Queer theory', *Group Analysis* 38, 67–81.

Chapter 3

Queer Family Therapy –
A Contradiction in Terms?

Alex Iantaffi

From a Journey to a Question

In September of 2002 I embarked on a journey to become a systemic family psychotherapist or, as this profession is more commonly known, a 'Marriage and Family Therapist'. At this point in my life I had already been an academic for some time, I had a PhD and I openly identified as queer. The course was not chosen lightly. This was the culmination of an even longer journey and was influenced by both lived experiences and deeply held epistemological beliefs. I chose a course heavily influenced by social constructionist approaches to therapy and that was explicitly welcoming of diversity. By the end of this journey, I was still pleased with that initial step but also aware of the painful turns in the path, often marked by encounters with an embedded heteronormativity, which I believe characterized not my course alone but seemingly the whole discipline, the whole field of therapy. This chapter portrays reflections on my journey but also on the journeys of some fellow travellers, which were collected as part of my dissertation research. The latter focused on the experiences of talking about sexual orientation within the context of a family therapy training course. In this chapter, as well as presenting the findings from my small and specific case study, I aim to raise the question of whether family therapy training can be truly queer-inclusive since its foundations lie on an heteronormative (and culturally specific) understanding of the concept of family. I will be using queer in the rest of this chapter as a term that I regard to be both more inclusive of non-heteronormative identities as well as to clearly indicate the influence that queer theory has had on those reflections.

In the previous paragraph, I mentioned social constructionism and, within this context, knowledge is seen as being historically, culturally and geographically specific as well as created and maintained through social processes (Burr, 1995). Adopting this position means that I view research as yet another social process whose aim it is, in my opinion, to open and participate in dialogue. Thus, as a researcher, I do not seek to uncover 'true' stories or to find the best way to integrate the dimension of sexuality in psychotherapy training, which would 'close off options for dialogue' (Gergen, 1999: 223), but merely to create a forum for new conversations and dialogues to emerge between the domains of queer theory and family therapy. In doing so, dogmatism is abandoned in favour of openness to the wider range of human experiences (Gergen, 1999). Furthermore, if I move from this position, reflexivity becomes an integral part of the research process, as well as being part of the training to become systemic family psychotherapists, especially in relation to the concept of growing 'into the identity of being a psychotherapist' (Hedges and Lang, 1993: 277). If knowledge is not 'out there', existing independently from relationships and interactions, waiting to be uncovered, or discovered, through the research process, but it is, instead, co-created (Shotter and Katz, 1998), then reflexivity is the ability that allows us to remain conscious co-creators throughout this process. In our everyday life we often are involved in 'a myriad of spontaneous, responsive, practical, unselfconscious, but contested interactions' (Shotter, 1993: 20), and reflexivity creates the space within us to be still and consider what social worlds and identities we are creating, for ourselves and each other, through our actions and interactions. This seems to be of particular importance within the context of family psychotherapy training, since, as therapist, we continuously invite families to explore their 'stories lived' and 'stories told' (Pearce, 1994) and often de-construct and re-construct these stories with them.

The importance of reflexivity was captured by the practice of 'mapping' in my training course, that is the opportunity for trainees to 'reflect on their work, reflect on their personal and professional identities; be "in the systemic client's chair"' (Hedges and Lang, 1993: 280). The latter system gave me plenty of opportunities to reflect on the intersectionality (Davis, 2008) of my queer identity and my budding experiences as a therapist, leading eventually to the question of whether there was space for queer experiences within family therapy training. Moving from this epistemological position also places my writing within the framework of autoethnographic methods (see Etherington, 2004 and Carolyn and Bochner, 2000). It is within this framework that I will try to weave a narrative whose threads are my story, the case studies, the existing literature and some reflections on the need for further exploration of the issues that emerge from this particular tapestry.

Family, Sexuality and How a New Journey Started

Growing up, I never questioned that I would have a husband and children, unless I decided to answer what I considered to be my vocation as a teenager and become a nun. For the first two decades of my life I lived in Italy and was raised in a Catholic culture, although other influences were also strongly present, such as my father's belief in communism, the power of trade unions and critical thinking. During this time, I never questioned my sexuality or indeed acknowledged the existence of sexual orientation. I was steeped in a heteronormative environment, representing a place in which heterosexuality is seen as the elemental form of human association, as the very model of inter-gender relations, as the indivisible basis of all community, and as the means of reproduction without which society would not exist (Warner, 1993: xxi).

The story of how I now come to identify as queer would probably fill the pages of an entirely different journey but suffice to say that this is how I identify now, both in relation to gender and sexual orientation. I believe parts of my story to be similar to those of other queer people since few of us had the luxury to consider that our identities were part of an acceptable spectrum of being. Just like many people who identify as something other than heterosexual, I have experienced for myself how others can express hatred towards you, without knowing you, just because of whom you are holding hands with or kiss on the lips. Because of these experiences I believe that my identity influences not just whom I happen to have sex with but how I see the world, others and myself. Therefore, my identity was certainly a factor when I decided to train with a specific institution since I felt that the course actively encouraged engaging with issues of diversity, for example by mentioning the GRRAACCEESS[1] in its literature. Nevertheless, I was not entirely surprised when sexuality seemed to be a rather unspoken facet of diversity. The papers we were asked to read on the subject were scarce (two in four years, in my case) and some of the discussions with my course mates difficult. I started to wonder whether I had been wise to choose family therapy, as surely the word family itself can indicate one particular way of seeing the world, through heteronormative lenses. Talking about sexual orientation on my course seemed to be something I could do only as an aside, in parenthesis. If I became too insistent, I found myself facing questions on whether I enjoyed being different, which had the effect to both divert us from considering the heterosexual privilege that seems pervasive in both the literature and the training, and to position my discomfort as a personal, rather than a political issue. Yet I started to wonder whether there were other trainees who felt as I did, regardless of their own sexual orientation. Undertaking the research element of the course gave me an opportunity to address my curiosity. Nevertheless, I was cautious of how such curiosity might be received by others. My caution was reduced whenever I talked to either tutors, other trainees or friends within the queer community. They all felt this was a worthwhile topic to approach and, in fact, when I nearly decided to explore something else, my best friend exclaimed: 'But you have to do this! It's important and not just for you.' To me, this was a reminder of my feminist mantra: the personal is political, whether this was purely my personal experience or not, I would not find out unless I explored it further. Thus, the seeds for this work were firmly planted.

Taking a Detour through the Literature

Unfortunately, even a cursory search of the literature confirmed that sexuality is indeed an aspect not often talked about in relation to therapeutic training, unless

---

1   The acronym GRRAACCEESS (Roper Hall, 1993) is often used on my training course to remind us to pay attention to the following areas of diversity: Gender, Race, Religion, Age, Ability, Culture, Class, Education, Ethnicity, Sexuality and Spirituality.

it is seen as pathology. For example, Malley and Tasker (1999) highlight how little attention has been paid to the discourse of sexual orientation within the field of family therapy. They mention their search of the literature on sexuality within family therapy publications and conclude that out of over 13,200 articles published between 1975 and 1995, only 77 mentioned sexual orientation (op cit. 6). The very limited presence of issues related to sexual orientation in the literature seems to imply that heteronormativity is as pervasive in the field of therapy as it still is in our society at large. This seems consistent with the idea of therapeutic encounters having the potential of taking place in a 'mirrored room', that is, a place in which those dominant discourses present in society are reflected back, through our interactions, the language we use and the beliefs we hold (Hare-Mustin, 1997). In fact, even the paper by Malley and Tasker (1999) addresses the issue of sexual orientation as being primarily related to clients. Unfortunately one of the rare pictures depicted in a book focusing on the experiences of queer therapists in practice (Davies and Neal, 1996) is still negative, as those therapists speak about their frequent encounters with homophobia in the workplace and how some theoretical models can also be perceived as homophobic, for example within the psychoanalytical paradigm.

Another issue arising from the literature is that often, when looking at sexual orientation, there seems to be a dichotomous construct of heterosexual – homosexual. For example, to use the Malley and Tasker (1999) paper again, the terms lesbians and gay men are the only ones in the title. A more fluid (dare I say queer?) construct of sexuality seems alien within psychotherapy, yet it has been increasingly advocated in other disciplines, such as sociology, particularly by queer authors themselves. The work of Judith Butler (1990) on disrupting the idea of gender as dichotomous is of particular significance in this field and it underlines the unavoidable relationship between gender and sexual orientations/identities whilst disrupting the causal link traditionally attributed to them. Butler sees gender as performance: not who we are but what we do. Our performances of identities in relation to gender and sexuality can, however, be seen as arising within dominant ideological frameworks, such as patriarchy and heteronormativity. Kitzinger (1989), for example, talks about how lesbian identities have been, and are, regulated through liberal humanism. The latter has been pervasive in our society and I have witnessed it first hand in many conversations both outside and within the context of psychotherapy training. This ideology of liberal humanism sees sexual identities as irrelevant to social discourse as they strive to normalize homosexuality by describing it 'as just a different lifestyle' (Simon, 1996). Much as it would be simpler to leave sexuality in the bedroom, the impossibility of separating the personal from the political is highlighted when looking at several small-scale studies that revealed in Britain, as many as one quarter to half of the population sampled, believed that it was 'unacceptable' for lesbians and gay men to have jobs that entailed dealing with the public (Snape et al., 1995). The recent recognition for same-sex partnerships through legal civil partnership in Britain is hopefully a sign that things have somewhat changed over the past decade yet it is also necessary to notice the resistance to this change by many members of the public.

Sexual orientation in therapy training also remains an issue, which is more or less relevant depending on the theoretical model followed. Davies and Neal (2000), for example, have written an extensive analytical account of how a range of models has considered the issue of homosexuality within a historical context, highlighting the difficulties that some of these models present for queer clients. Furthermore, more recently Milton and Coyle (2003: 488) reported how a psychoanalytical therapy trainee felt that 'the therapist wasn't going to pass a trainee who was a practising gay man'. Besides acceptance by tutors or clinical supervisors, queer trainees can also feel alienated by theoretical models who implicitly exclude them by focusing on purely heteronormative discourses, such as the Family Life Cycle model (Carter and McGoldrick, 1989). Such exclusions can compound the institutional silences, such as lack of a significant number of papers on the topic, lack of reference to one's own identity in equal opportunities policies, which usually mention gay men and lesbians but not bisexuals and transgender people. This void of reference points can lead queer trainees to feel not valued or out of place and, when resisting such a void, to find themselves isolated and disappointed, as the person who always brings up the issue (Coyle et al., 1999). Reading the literature, I found myself reflecting on those moments when I have also felt isolated and disappointed. Yet I also held a strong belief that adopting a social constructionist stance, which my course in systemic therapy seemed to do, created the possibility for dialogue on these issues. My curiosity created a context for a neutral stance, 'in a commitment to evolving differences, with a concomitant nonattachment to any particular position' (Cecchin, 1987: 406).

The web of relationships, between my own stories, those of others around me and the ideas presented by the literature, led me to formulate some research questions, which I used as a further compass throughout this particular research journey:

- What stories do we tell about sexuality within the context of systemic family psychotherapy training?
- What stories of sexuality do we, as trainee family psychotherapists, live and which of these stories do we choose to tell both in the classroom and in clinical practice?

Shared Landscapes

When I decided to interview other family therapy students within my institution, I wanted the interviews to be safe spaces, where participants could share their experiences of being a trainee, and talk about themselves and others on the course, through the lens of sexuality. This safety needed to encompass the relational aspect too by, for instance, ensuring that the conversational space allowed people to express their identities, feel validated and, most importantly, not to feel judged (MacNeil and Mead, 2005). All these factors led me to choose individual case studies (Gomm and Hammersley, 2000; Yin, 1989), and to have in-depth conversations which allowed me to listen more intently both to them and myself (Burck, 2005; Reinharz, 1992). From the analysis of these conversations, some generative themes emerged (Freire, 1972), which, when compared and combined with those of other participants, created a 'thematic universe' unique to their particular group. This 'universe' of themes was then contrasted and compared with the existing literature and the methodological framework.

Five generative themes in particular emerged as central to all those conversations:

- the place of sexuality on the training course;
- safety;
- positions;
- the differences that would make the difference;
- reflecting on the research process.

Each theme was also connected to several sub-themes, connected to each other, creating a web of relationships across themes but it would be impossible to fully report on my findings in this chapter, therefore, in this section, I will try to give an overview of the major themes, using the participants' voices as much as possible.

Both case studies' participants, Anna and Sarah,[2] talked extensively about the place that sexuality seems to hold in our training programme. This covered several aspects of the course, ranging from practical aspects, such as the small number of papers dedicated to the subject, to more theoretical ones, such as the impact of training within social constructionist framework. Talking about the former, Anna stated:

> My experience has been that sexuality has really been either completely invisible or if there's actually a paper on the reading list, it's the only paper about sexuality in year four and it's on the optional reading list. I know that now there's been ... I've noticed a couple of workshops coming out, there's one on queer theory coming up and there was one quite recently about working with gay clients or something ... So that was kind of like, "Oh my god, how amazing", but I was quite curious about who would go to those as well, whether you were actually just preaching to the converted.

Similar feelings were shared by Sarah who talked of the small number of papers on sexuality as a 'glaring omission, because of my special interest'. The number of papers on sexuality included in the syllabus, as well as the workshops in this area listed in our institution's programme seemed to create a context, for both

---

2   Please note that the name of the participants have been changed to ensure confidentiality and anonymity.

participants, which did not seem to be welcoming of this particular diversity. This was a feeling I also shared and both conversations veered, at different points, towards the discussion of the model used to invite reflection on social diversity, that is the GRRAACCEESS. Sarah talked about feeling that sexuality 'is sort of the silent S' in this model. This was not only due to her experiences on the course but also to knowing a graduate with whom she has had a difficult conversation, as illustrated by her words below.

> I feel that because it seems to receive less attention during the course, people are graduating from the course without sufficient awareness, I suppose, of the issues. I've had conversations with one graduate from the course who seemed to have ideas that I would have hoped not to find in a systemic therapist, I suppose, prejudices about different people with, well, non heterosexual people, let's put it that way, yeah. (…) Quite strong ideas, which I don't find very systemic or very therapeutic.

Anna also talked about the GRRAACCEESS and felt that, as a model, they had the potential to close dialogues off, rather than opening them. She also felt that it could lead to what I have defined as a hierarchy of oppression, especially with other people on the course who fell into other categories of minority grouping. This idea was present in both conversations and is illustrated by Anna's words as quoted below.

> We would often talk about frustrations but between us there was almost this kind of rivalry about whether there was a hierarchy or not, so actually it didn't feel supportive, because I felt like when I was saying, yes, sexuality, it was like: yeah, but that's not the same and this is actually more important. (…) But you can't have a hierarchy of the GRRAACCEESS, that's ridiculous, because actually people are getting killed still from queer bashing and people don't get jobs and there's so much discrimination and prejudice and you can't say that that is somehow less. And again this other person would say, "But you have a choice whether you choose to disclose" and I said, "Oh, so you're recommending to stay in the closet then, because otherwise you're not safe". And that used to drive me insane. But you're somehow having to find a way of validating your position or justifying your position.

As the conversations unfolded, I felt that my participants seemed to share what I too found to be a paradox in my training. The GRRAACCEESS were seen as positioning us in boxes that were not spacious or connected enough and seemed to have little value beyond the mnemonic acronym. On the one hand, all three of us had chosen this course because of its theoretical framework; on the other our weekly experiences did not reflect the constructionist nature of our course. Sarah talked about how:

When I came to consider the course it resonated with me, because I think I've always been a social constructionist before I knew the term. From a young ... from my teens really, I've had the view that a lot of issues of social differences, well, all issues of social difference are socially constructed and therefore I would have expected the course to follow that through.

Anna also chose the course because of its emphasis on social constructionism and, despite her negative experiences, she talked about how the theories studied offered her a lens through which to make sense of them:

I think I'm much more mindful about group dynamics and the whole idea of positioning theory and inviting people into certain ways and resisting certain things and what power do you have to be able to do that. So, I suppose using the theory as well has been quite exciting.

I am mindful that this quote was within the context of Anna feeling isolated from her peer group and often taking an observer position. Nevertheless, theory was definitely an aspect of the course that seemed to permeate several of the themes brought up in the conversations, almost as a thread running through them, in fact. As well as social constructionism and positioning theory, neutrality and curiosity were also aspects of systemic practice that were mentioned in relation to sexual orientation. Sarah talked about how better awareness of one's prejudices:

Is not a question of knowledge, it's a question of, I suppose, it's a question of a way of thinking that allows us to be, in lay terms, open minded or um, you might call it curious um about anybody who might walk into our therapy rooms. That we have developed the ability not to make any assumptions and to remain curious whatever we're told about that person.

Unfortunately, as Anna stated:

I think systemic therapy and social construction therapy are there so how I've used them has been brilliant, but I think in the training context they're taught in a very specific way, which is a very heterosexual way, kind of thing.

I found myself sharing with the participants a sense that our training ran the same risk, highlighted for a therapeutic context, to become a 'mirrored room'. Similar feelings are echoed by Sarah who also stated that:

It felt like quite a reflection of the issue of sexuality in society in a way, ... the way it is a kind of invisible, ... very often, ... invisible sort of aspect of life for people and a high degree of marginalization of LGB people, it felt that was kind of reflected within the training context. (...) I've heard some clichés and some stereotyping remarks from both tutors and other trainees. Sometimes said jokingly but I'm not sure even that's appropriate. (...) I felt defensive because it's kind of confirmed for me the position of sexual minorities in society, if you like, and I think, well, if tutors and students are thinking and speaking like this, then the general public must be speaking and thinking in ways which are more damaging and more marginalizing and just have more preconceived ideas, misconceptions, whatever.

Another thread emerging from the conversations was that of the role of the tutors. Both the issue of training reflecting the prejudices of society, by being a mirrored room, and this issue are closely linked to how safe the participants had felt on the course, in relation to issues of sexual orientation. Positioning themselves as people who were interested in issues of sexual orientation seemed to have an impact on the degree of safety, which they experienced with both tutors and fellow trainees. The way in which tutors interacted with participants in relation to issues of sexual orientation was varied, which also reflected my experiences. On the one hand both the participants and myself have worked with people who did not seem to have much awareness, whilst on the other, some were able to engage with the issue in a different way, as shown in the following quotations:

[When talking about LGBT clients], I was shocked and dismayed by how they were talked about, not just by other trainees, but by the supervisor as well and I was furious and disgusted and surprised and lots of different things, so I suppose that really informs me as well in terms of oh my god, you're having to really start at the real basics. (...) I think the [other] tutor has thought a lot about sexuality because she's worked with some lesbian and gay clients and I think one of her supervisor's is a lesbian but she's not herself. And I think because she was there, I don't know, people were behaving themselves, I don't know, but it was really lovely to sit back and watch to the point that after we'd been going on for about fifteen minutes I said, I really love that I'm at XXX and that we're talking seriously about cottaging, fantastic! (Anna)

I think it's also happened in other ways that students have expressed ideas that don't really have a place in a systemic therapy training and my expectation of a tutor would be that they would deal with that, that they would, you know, explore those ideas with the student and make sure they didn't position any other trainees in a way that was marginalizing or threatening or anything, but that, for some reasons, isn't what tutors do. I would say somebody like X and maybe Y do display a kind of ... an ability, more of an ability to kind of take a stance of not knowing, if you like and I don't feel I would ever hear anything marginalizing or stereotyping from them. At the same time I don't think either of them have probably really explored the issues, would really know what might be the experience of a non heterosexual client in their therapy room. (Sarah)

The range of tutors and their attitudes seemed to have an effect on the participants feeling safe enough to tackle issues of sexuality, as it depends on

> Who's in the room at the time, in a way, um because I feel that the thing that makes the difference is particular individuals. (...) I guess I worry about being judged. (Sarah)

Anna talked about how she never felt quite safe enough on the course as to bring her personal stories, both during social time, such as breaks, or course time:

> I don't think I've ever spoken 100% of myself and felt safe, well, I've never done it. It would feel like I was putting myself under scrutiny if I did that and I think I'd be worried I'd have to justify or validate myself or explain things and I just haven't had the energy to do that and I haven't felt that it would actually make a difference if I did, because I'm just one voice in an heterosexual, dominant culture. (...) I think that's been a really big difference the whole course is when we've talked about what's informed our questions or whatever, I have always drawn on my professional identity and whereas other people say, "Well as a mother of a fifteen-year old or as someone who's been married for twenty-five years" ... or whatever it may be ... and I don't.

Like myself, the other trainees found safe spaces outside the course to talk about their experiences and frustrations:

> It actually felt most comfortable talking about it at work and I talked a lot and often by taking the piss out of it, saying oh god, you won't believe what happened yesterday. So often I'm not so angry when I talk about it here [at work], but it's a way of diffusing it and then people might be angry and say, I can't believe that happened! So people get angry with me and I'm like, yeah and stuff like that, so I kind of get my validity here. Validity about my anger and my shock that people think like this, I mean I think that's the biggest thing, that, oh my god, they're still out there! (Anna)

Stereotypes, hurtful positioning and remarks, are 'still out there' and appeared to contribute greatly to the participants feeling unsafe at times. Therefore the awareness, or lack of it, on the course, was a theme that came up consistently. For example, Sarah shares her experience of meeting a tutor during an assessment and highlights what took place:

> I'm not really talking about knowledge here, but more of a question of awareness, that I had much greater awareness than he did and that seems the wrong way around, it seemed inappropriate. (...) I felt this was the first time he'd ever thought about it, I distinctly got that impression and that made me feel a bit unsafe.

Later, however, she also acknowledges that things are changing, when she states 'I think perhaps it is happening, just a bit slowly but maybe it'll get there, it will get better'.

Anna also frames the issue of awareness within the wider context of our training being focused on family therapy:

> I think because, um, you know, family therapy is often talked about and I think "family" in family therapy is still heterosexual and that's after events I've been to, you know, where it doesn't get mentioned and from lots of other contexts that it's as if it doesn't exist, lesbian and gay lifestyles and, if they do, they're this weird freaky exception.

Such lack of awareness, as well as making the participants feel unsafe, also influences the position they choose to take, or feel cornered into taking, often through fear of being marginalized because of their sexual identity or passion about sexuality issues:

> I think I was concerned that that [personal stories and professional interest in relation to sexuality] could go against me as well, that in, for instance, giving a presentation that aimed to increase awareness of the issue, I might also be, that my very ideas and my presentation and I myself might be marginalized because of the subject matter ... (Sarah)

I felt I shared this complex dance of positioning with both participants, although we all found ourselves in a variety of situations and dancing different steps. The positions adopted by both participants varied, both throughout the conversations, and in the stories they told me about their experiences of training. Both Sarah and Anna talked about positioning themselves, within the contexts described so far, as well as feeling positioned by others in particular ways. They talked about feeling positioned as champions, pioneers or crusaders, yet they responded to such positioning in different ways. Sarah initially talks about how experiencing the training context as a reflection of society's prejudices made her feel positioned as a 'champion of the cause', which she embraced to a degree, but she also reflected on the context that influenced such positioning:

> In some ways it's kind of helped me become a champion, because I've felt that there was a kind of blank page for me to make my mark, if you like. Um, there was new ground for me to break, if I'd felt my particular cause I wanted to champion was, um, let's think, culture and race say, then I'd feel I was simply following a lot of other people and would find it much more difficult to make my own mark, whereas this way I felt that almost anything I did would be kind of different and further the existing awareness on the course, um, so it was a kind of positive in a way. But at the same time I wondered how it positioned me, would I be marginalized? (...) So it was kind of two edged (...) I think the reason I've felt positioned as I have, you know, as a bit of a crusader, is for a reason and

the reason is that, um, there's been a crusade to fight and I don't think I'd have imagined that. I didn't position myself that way, without the system being in place for that to happen.

Anna also talked about how she felt positioned by the training context. Some of the experiences of supervision, as described earlier in this chapter, positioned her within the group as challenging and she then felt invited, by her tutors, to adopt a position of staying 'silent on issues of sexuality'. This invitation was met with anger on her part, as explained below in her own words:

> I think for me the anger was about the fact that you're in a minority position as someone who has a minority sexuality, however you choose to define that and you're being told to keep quiet about it, you're being oppressed, heterosexuality is being privileged because it's making people feel uncomfortable. And I do agree that there are certain ways that you can talk about it, but actually sometimes you need to directly challenge people as well and I think it's also something about not being validated, both as a person but also, I think, from your life experience. (...) I've got so much experience that I could have brought into this course and it's just not been invited, actually, which is not my loss, because I'm fine, thank you very much, but then to be told to actually, can you keep the tiny bits you show quiet, because I'm not showing them in the right way, it just felt, well, do you want me to coat everything in sugar? It just felt horribly oppressive and having no sense of awareness that what you're doing is not ok.

Other people can also be seen as positioning us. In the case of Anna, her feeling of oppression seemed compounded by fellow trainees adopting a position of undisputed entitlement when openly discussing their heterosexual lifestyles:

> Everyone else in the group has children and they always talk about it every week, they always talk about children and it gets brought into, it reflects the team conversations and whatever and they started to annoy me a bit because, as someone who has always wanted children (...) Well, it was a really big issue for me for a long time and so I actually felt, you're all in a really privileged position that, by being heterosexual, it's just so straightforward to you and you have no awareness of the privilege you're speaking from. I tried to explain that and nobody got it at all and I think they thought I was being supersensitive or something, I don't know, I don't know ...

This lack of awareness ultimately led Anna to adopting an observer position, but it also made her feel positioned as an expert:

> Because it's almost like you have to step out of the trainee role and say, "Right, we're going to talk about sexuality now and I'm going to get the conversation going". But actually I'd like to be a trainee and do it. Because I think when you

step out of the trainee role and then you're the expert on it, you're not learning anymore, apart from how to say things in a gentle way, without being clear, do you know what I mean? Whereas if the course was owning it, then you could come and say, well, these are my ideas and how do they fit and not feel worried that people are going to invalidate your experience and say, well, that doesn't count because it's not heterosexual!

This dance of mutual positioning seems to interact with the acceptability of different issues of social diversity, as already highlighted when discussing the GRRAACCEESS.

I think what's fascinating is that this is a training where you're meant to be self-reflective and think about all the parts of your identity but it's almost like some parts are more welcome than others, because the ones that are maybe minority parts make other people feel uncomfortable. Why, I don't know, because maybe they don't get it, I don't know what it is, but they're having to think about what that means, if you position yourself in a minority, they have to position themselves in a majority and maybe that's hard to think about. (Anna)

Reflecting on how these positions were being influenced by the various contexts present in training, such as own and other people's experiences, the tutors, the papers and clients' cases, led me to ask future oriented questions to explore what could be done differently during training for the issue of sexuality to be positioned differently.

Envisioning Different Possibilities

Some of the stories shared so far might seem quite negative, yet there were also exceptions and, as well as exploring them, Sarah, Anna and I talked about what could be different in our training in order for us to feel things are as we would wish them to be, in relation to the issue of sexual orientation. Both participants talked about how some small changes, such as more reading material on the topic in the syllabus, would make them feel quite differently about the training, as they would create a different context from which to speak, whilst also acknowledging that some of these changes have already started:

I think there was the realization that it wasn't until the third year that there was a single workshop about any form of sexuality, um, but what's interesting is that now, in the fourth year, that's increased 100% and there are two workshops on sexuality, so to me that kind of confirms that it needed to change. In a way it makes me think maybe something's been taken on board about the protests that we've made about the lack of inclusion of that, yeah. (…) I mean I would love to think that um it would all be taken on board, you know, if you come out with something that does suggest that certain things could be done differently, like (…) that next year's reading list for all years was more inclusive and that, to me, would indicate that the thinking had shifted, something concrete and tangible. (Sarah)

I think if the course actually had some ownership on talking about sexuality, so it didn't feel like it was me bringing it, so if they had stuff on the reading list, if they had dedicated time, this next few weeks we're going to be thinking about sexuality in all its many forms and what are our own ideas and feelings about it. Then I'd be able to be a participant with everyone else and say what my thoughts are from my own life experience. (…) Yes, it's about ownership, I think it's about the course saying, well, it's important to talk about, you need to take this seriously, we're going to help you do that, we're going to put it on the curriculum, you know, this is something that should be integrated throughout your training, for you to think about as another social difference. (…) It's about really having it, I think, central to your organization where you do have lesbian and gay staff. Why not have the Gay Times on the papers table next to Hello magazine in reception. Have lesbian and gay books on the shelves, have, you know, regular workshops about it, you know, just have it as a presence that's there, that's not made into something unusual or different or special, but it's just kind of there without having to even think about it. (Anna)

Such concrete changing, such as talking about sexuality and including more papers about the topic, would also lead to a greater sense of safety according to Sarah, as well as bringing a sense of increased awareness about the issue. In a similar vein, Anna saw increased awareness as something that would happen if lesbian and gay staff were employed by the organization, or at least,

… staff that worked in lesbian and gay, or with lesbian and gay clients, they don't have to be lesbian and gay themselves but actually were more aware of the issues themselves. It would just be brought in naturally, rather than having to make a big song and dance about it.

She also mentioned that lesbian and gay mentors, available for all trainees, regardless of their sexual orientation, would make a difference.

Many of the differences mentioned by the participants connected with my desire to also shift the focus of sexuality from the personal to the political. As Anna, states, this was not an issue that was purely personal to her either.

I think it is feeling validated but I think it's almost like not just personally validated. But I almost feel like I'm the one who's flying the rainbow flag and it's for the cause that it should be validated, so it's all the gay clients that I work with it should be validated. It's for my friends it should be validated. It's for the wider community it should be validated and I think on one level it is personal validation but I think on the wider level, because my views are just mine (...). I think if it came from the course there'd be more space for having, within sexuality, all the different, you know, you have right wing lesbian and gay people, as well as left wing lesbian and gay people, and to have all that space, whereas if it just comes from me, you just get left with feminist kind of sexuality.

As the conversations unfolded and as I revisited them, it became clear to me that the personal was the political for Anna and Sarah. In some ways I found myself where I started but with a broader view of the landscape, which obviously extended beyond the confines of my individual training journey. Once I identified patterns in the data and organized it in the five generative themes mentioned earlier, I also started to see connections to the literature on the topic, which I had considered at the beginning of this journey. It could be argued that the literature itself had been one of my maps and, as such, I only found the landmarks that I expected to find. However, I believe that the method and techniques used left much room for my travelling companions to show me what they noticed in the landscape, as well as me pointing out a few landmarks with my questions. The value of this account and my connections are for the readers to judge and I have hopefully been transparent enough about the journey so that they can do that.

The experiences of Anna and Sarah seem to reflect some of the themes in the literature. Just as Malley and Tasker (1999) pointed out that little attention had been given to issues of sexual orientation on paper, within the field of family therapy, so it seems to be also in practice, within the context of training. The place of sexuality on the training course was, in fact, one of the most extensive generative themes presented. This included various aspects of the course from the more concrete, such as the number of papers in the reading list or the books on the shelves in our institution, to the less tangible, such as the level of awareness of both tutors and trainees. The stories told during these conversations seem, unfortunately, to reflect existing accounts of therapists encountering homophobia within the work context (Davies and Neal, 1996). The training context, in the stories that have unfolded on this journey, can be seen as just another 'mirrored room' (Hare-Mustin, 1997), in which our society's homophobic attitudes (Snape et al., 1995) are still present. Both Sarah and Anna realized that this cannot be avoided. After all trainees and tutors are co-creators of this society too. Yet, like me, they longed for different interactions, in the hope that these might change the context in which we move.

Their hope and longing, like mine, was influenced by the theoretical ideas promoted on our training course. They also believed that not all theoretical approaches are compatible with a non-heteronormative outlook, as pointed out in the literature (Davies and Neal, 2000) and chose a specific course because of its commitment to a social constructionist outlook. Furthermore, both Anna and Sarah saw the potential of the tools of this framework, such as mapping (Hedges and Lang, 1993), to increase both their own and other people's ability to be reflexive. Nevertheless, they often felt steeped in a culture of 'liberal humanism' (Kitzinger, 1989) where sexuality could be seen just as an element of one's personal lifestyle (Simon, 1996) rather than a collective, powerful discourse. Such personalization of the issue, combined with the lack of concrete reference points, indicating the organization's lack of ownership of this topic, led both participants to fear and feel marginalized, isolated and/or positioned as champions or experts, which often led to them feeling silenced. These positions and feelings were also present in the literature reviewed (Coyle et al., 1999), which, together with the participants' words, seem to call for a closer, more political and fearless relationship between sexuality and psychotherapy training. This could be achieved, as pointed out by Anna and Sarah when exploring the difference that would make the difference, by changing both higher contexts and actions. For example, social constructionism, the idea of therapy as a cybernetic of prejudices (Cecchin et al., 1994) and relational reflexivity (Burnham 2005) can exercise a contextual force for challenging both tutors' and trainees' homophobia. On the other hand, the concrete actions suggested, such as increasing the presence of issues of sexuality in the curriculum, or employing staff who identify and/or have experience of working with queer clients, could exercise a strong implicative force on widening the application of our theoretical frameworks to the issue of sexuality.

Future Journeys

Just like this particular journey has started with a small step, taken by myself a long time ago, this account could be seen as an invitation for training organizations to take that first step towards acknowledging the much wider range of human sexuality, which goes well beyond the dichotomy of male or female (Butler, 1990), especially when adopting a social constructionist position. This would not just be a personal act towards the individual trainees who have spoken out on this journey. It would be, as they themselves have said, a political act of challenging homophobia in all its forms, and by so doing validating the experiences of both queer trainees and clients. Such an act, albeit radical, entails small deeds, such as the ones suggested by the participants themselves: the inclusion of a wider range of papers about sexuality in the syllabus; the literature on display in the premises used; the seminars offered to both students and qualified therapists; the employment of tutors who are both able and willing to engage with discourses about sexuality. This radical act is, however, also composed by larger deeds, which require an ongoing commitment to challenging heteronormative discourses within the field of systemic therapy. These larger deeds would include, for example, challenging traditional definitions of family and models, such as that of the family life cycle. They would also include the use of practices already in existence, like mapping, to create safe spaces in which a wider breadth of diversity, including different sexualities, can be expressed without fear of being invalidated by either tutors or peers. Such deeds would not happen overnight but the smaller ones would at least start a repositioning of our field. This shift seems to have been long overdue, in relation to issues about sexuality, if the latter is to move from its current place in parenthesis to a more central position that allows for new stories to be lived and told by future trainees. Looking at my position at the end of this particular journey, it can be seen as quite similar to the one I started from. I am still an out queer person in the world, a systemic therapist who became licensed in the UK and is now undergoing the licensure process in the US, a feminist, a social constructionist and a researcher. Once again, reflexivity is the thread running through this journey and, therefore, it seems apt to punctuate the end of this account with some personal reflections.

On a personal level, I have come to better appreciate the forces that can be set in motion by my decision not to be closeted about aspects of my identity, whilst also respecting other people's different positioning. There are so many stories and conversations influencing such a choice for each individual that it would once again take a separate chapter and a much broader research project to explore them all. However, for the purposes of this story told by me to you, it is worth highlighting that some of my own stories have changed. When I took that first step on the course I felt scared, anxious and informed by a desire to be liked by everyone around me. Having taken this journey I must admit to no longer feeling the latter. Being out as queer is still scary and worrying at times but I accept that, for some people, liking me for who I am is a bigger challenge than what they are able to tolerate from their current position. I also feel freer in choosing my own positions and ability to reflect on which opportunities that openness about my sexual identity can bring, as well as considering which opportunities might be closed down by it. In this context the personal is still political but both the personal and political are constructs created in the interactions of which I am part. It is therefore worth asking myself, each time, 'What do I want to co-create? and which position would it be most useful to speak from in this situated moment'. I believe this to be particularly important as a systemic therapist and researcher, since my choice to be open/closed about my sexual orientation will create more or less useful therapeutic encounters and fruitful research journeys.

Finally, I believe that it is now time for a more open debate in the field of family therapy about where we go next. Creating new models to box the lives of lesbians and gay men is no longer satisfactory as heteronormative discourses can still be pervasive in these models. I believe, instead, that it is time to embrace the possibilities offered by discourses such as queer theory and by the lived experiences of those of us who choose to identify as more fluid in our sexuality and gender, thus refusing to fit into easier labels and models.

References

Burck, C. (2005), 'Comparing qualitative research methodologies for systemic research: The use of grounded theory, discourse analysis and narrative analysis', *Journal of Family Therapy* 27, 237–262.

Burnham, J. (2005), 'Relational reflexivity: A tool for socially constructing therapeutic relationships', in Flaskas C., Mason, B. and Perlesz, A. (eds), *The Space Between: Experience, Context and Process in the Therapeutic Relationship* (London: Karnac Books).

Burr, V. (1995), *An Introduction to Social Constructionism* (London: Routledge).

Butler, J. (1990), *Gender Trouble: Feminism and the Subversion of Identity* (London: Routledge).

Carolyn, E. and Bochner, A.P. (2000), 'Autoethnography, personal narrative, reflexivity: Researcher as subject', in Denzin, N. and Lincoln, Y. (eds), *The Handbook of Qualitative Research* (2nd Edition) (Thousand Oaks, CA: Sage), pp. 733–768.

Carter, B. and McGoldrick, M. (1989), *The Changing Family Life Cycle: A Framework for Family Therapy* (London: Gardner Press).

Cecchin, G. (1987), 'Hypothesizing, circularity, and neutrality revisited: An invitation to curiosity', *Family Process* 26(4), 405–413.

Cecchin, G., Lane, G. and Ray, W.A. (1994), *The Cybernetics of Prejudices in the Practice of Psychotherapy* (London: Karnac Books).

Coyle, A., Milton M. and Annesley P. (1999), 'The silencing of lesbian and gay voices in psychotherapeutic texts and training', *Changes: An International Journal of Psychology and Psychotherapy* 17, 132–143.

Davies, D. and Neal, C. (eds) (1996), *Pink Therapy* (Buckingham: Oxford University Press).

Davies, D. and Neal, C. (eds) (2000), *Pink Therapy 2: Therapeutic Perspectives on Working with Lesbian, Gay and Bisexual Clients* (Buckingham: Open University Press).

Davis, K. (2008), 'Intersectionality as buzzword. A sociology of science perspective on what makes a feminist theory successful', *Feminist Theory* 9(1), 67–85.

Etherington, K. (2004), *Becoming a Reflexive Researcher: Using Our Selves in Research* (London: Jessica Kingsley Publishers).

Freire, P. (1972), *Pedagogy of the Oppressed* (Middlesex: Penguin Education).

Gergen, K.J. (1999), *An Invitation to Social Construction* (London: Sage).

Gomm, R., Hammersley M. and Foster P. (eds) (2000), *Case Study Method* (London: Sage).

Hare-Mustin, R.T. (1997), 'Discourse in the mirrored room. A post-modern analysis of therapy', in Gergen M.M. and Davis S.N. (eds), *Toward a New Psychology of Gender. A Reader* (London: Routledge), pp. 553–574.

Hedges, F. and Lang, S. (1993), 'Mapping personal and professional stories', *Human Systems* 4, 277–298.

Kitzinger, C. (1989), 'The regulation of lesbian identities: Liberal humanism as an ideology of social control', in Shotter, J. and Gergen, K.J. (eds), *Texts of Identity* (London: Sage), pp. 82–98.

MacNeil, C. and Mead, S. (2005), 'A narrative approach to developing standards for trauma-informed peer support', *American Journal of Evaluation* 26(2), 231–244.

Malley, M. and Tasker, F. (1999), 'Lesbians, gay men and family therapy: A contradiction in terms?', *Journal of Family Therapy* 21, 3–29.

Milton, M. and Coyle, A. (2003), 'Sexual identity: Affirmative practices with lesbian and gay clients', in Wolfe, R., Dryden, W. and Strawbridge, S. (eds), *Handbook of Counselling Psychology* (2nd Edition) (London: Sage).

Pearce, W.B. (1994), *Interpersonal Communication: Making Social Worlds* (London: HarperCollins).

Reinharz, S. (1992), *Feminist Methods in Social Research* (Oxford: Oxford University Press).

Roper Hall, A. (1993), cited in Burnham, J. 'Systemic supervision: The evolution of reflexivity in the context of the supervisory relationship', *Human Systems* 4, 349–381.

Shotter, J. (1993), *Conversational Realities* (London: Sage).

Shotter, J. and Katz, A.M. (1998), 'Creating relational realities. Responsible responding to poetic "movements" and "moments"', in McNamee, S. and Gergen, K.J. (eds), *Relational Responsibility: Resources for Sustainable Dialogue* (London: Sage), pp. 151–161.

Simon, G. (1996), 'Working with people in relationships', in Davies, D. and Neal, C. (eds), *Pink Therapy* (Buckingham: Oxford University Press).

Snape, D., Thompson, K. and Chetwynd, M. (1995), *Discrimination Against Gay Men and Lesbians: A Study of the Nature and Extent of Discrimination Against Homosexual Men and Women in Britain Today* (London: Social and Community Planning Research).

Warner, M. (1993), 'Introduction', in Warner, M. (ed.), *Fear of a Queer Planet: Queer Politics and Social Theory* (Minneapolis: University of Minnesota Press).

Yin, R.K. (1989), *Case Study Research: Design and Methods* (Revised Edition) (Newbury Park, CA: Sage).

Chapter 4

Towards a Queer Praxis:
The Democratization of Feeling

Lyndsey Moon

This chapter calls for a democratization of feeling in relation to sex, sexuality and gender and the way this is configured via emotion words and concepts within the therapeutic arena. In this chapter, there is 'a rallying cry for collective action' (Lewis 2008, 74) to reconsider the language of emotion used to describe feelings. The chapter calls for a 'democratic imaginary' (Lewis 2008) leading to a full scale 'democratization' of feeling promoting the freedom, expression and description of feelings away from heteronormative meanings. It is primarily a 'stepping back' from the illogicality of emotion and the way it is presently attributed to real or imagined bodily 'feeling', how it is reflexively assigned to sexed, gendered and sexualized bodies and the way it acts as social capital in the structure of personhood and identity. It suggests instead that 'feeling', the ephemeral and ineffable quality of the corporeal body, is moved centre stage and re-evaluated as a main liberatory tool to bring about change in therapeutic meanings of sex, genders and sexualities. Rather than being assigned meaning through 'emotion' words and concepts that are shaped through the language of heteronormativity (in therapy this may be via numerous psychological texts that mention gender or sexuality including ICD and DSM[1]) which then structures knowledge about personhood and identity, in this chapter feeling, and in particular sexual feeling, is reappraised as a phenomena that can radically alter individual and collective meanings of emotion in relation to the gendered, sexed and sexualized body. Within queer communities, it seems as though feeling, including erotic/sexual feeling or 'erotic desire' (Valentine 2006) is consciously disengaged from the fixity of sexual, sexed and/or gendered identity. This allows for the reconfiguration of meanings for feelings, including sexual feelings, which then challenge normative structures.

---

1   The International Classification of Diseases (ICD) and Diagnostic and Statistical Manual (DSM) are used by virtually all psychologists as a sort of mental health dictionary of disordered thinking, behaviour and feeling. They describe numerous coded categories of mental illness i.e. disordered emotions and, until 1973 the DSM included homosexuality, until lobbying groups and social movements pressurized for this to be removed. The question of how a 'mental illness' can be removed en masse still requires much more explanation. The next version, DSM V is due out in 2012.

Previous research (Moon 2002) discovered a major disjuncture between emotion and feeling, with the naming of feeling through emotion words and concepts mediating the relationship of the individual and society. In fact, I suggested that emotion words/concepts and feeling may be referred to as objects[2] forming a 'system of meaning' (Blumer 1969) cognitively arranged or 'framed' (Goffman 1974) within the interaction. On the one hand social actors name their real or imagined bodily 'feeling states' through emotion words (e.g. I feel … angry, sad, happy etc.), while on the other hand society and culture give meaning to emotion words and concepts and these are assigned onto and into the body through a reflexive process and according to given social contexts. Feelings and their constituent emotion words and concepts basically tell us if we are 'in-line' (co-ordinated) with socially shared meanings about emotions, as well as how we interpret (co-orient) information in relation to socially organized meanings about emotion. It is a constant reflexive process. In this chapter I am suggesting that there is a place within therapy to consider the interaction between emotion and feeling as one that is representative of the way social meanings (emotion words and concepts) are reflexively assigned to the real or imagined 'feelings' of the social actor and then implicated in the ongoing construction of personhood. For this reason, I interrogate my most recent theoretical findings (Moon 2009) through the works of Pierre Bourdieu (1977) who argues through his discussion of 'field' and 'habitus' that 'the objective and subjective aspects of social life are inescapably bound together' (Marshall 1994, 8). For Bourdieu, the meaning of

---

2   According to Blumer (1969, 68–70), in Symbolic Interactionism all objects are social constructs and are anything that can be designated or referred to. According to Blumer (1969), an object is: 1) constituted by the meaning it has for the person for whom it is an object; 2) this meaning is not intrinsic to the object but arises from how the person is initially prepared to act towards it; 3) all objects are social products in that they are formed and transformed by the defining process that takes place in social interaction; 4) that people are prepared or set to act toward objects on the basis of the meaning of the objects for them; 5) just because an object is something that is designated, one can organize one's action toward it instead of responding immediately to it. My research suggested that feeling and emotions are discrete but strongly interlinked. Feelings are understood as 'abstract objects' while emotion word/concepts are understood as 'social objects' and in this scenario both feeling and emotions may be referred to or designated. Quite often, this means they are mistakenly understood as one and the same which is why most theorists in the study of emotion refer to feelings as emotions and vice versa. However, by locating feeling and emotion as separate objects it is possible to see how we socially construct meanings for emotions which we then assign to feeling states. My research found that the naming of feeling for self and other via emotion words/concepts is socially organized depending on context e.g. sexual identity, gender etc which is also constructed through social meanings in given contexts. Thus, emotion and feeling have their social meanings reflexively organized to the point where they become one and the same thing when in fact, their meanings need to be separated. For this reason, I have turned to the idea of habitus as that place where emotion and feeling represent a socialized subjectivity and subjective sociality.

objectivity and subjectivity is not a clear cut division. For him, the social is always shaping meanings and the social actor reflexively orders these meanings in relation to the habitus they are part of and at the same time, is part of them. The habitus is a 'socialized subjectivity' (Corber and Valocchi 2003) to the point that whatever we do or say, our actions and our words are always influenced by the social and influence the social at one and the same time. It is re-iterative ongoing process added to by reflexivity, as 'inner dialogue' or 'silent speech' (Archer 2003, 65) that acts a process of mediation through which agents use 'properties and powers [which are] distinct from those pertaining to social forms ... such as thinking, deliberating, believing, intending, loving and so forth which are applicable to people but never to social structures or cultural systems' (2003, 2).

Extending the notion of 'emotional habitus', defined as that place where culture has 'provided a language and a set of practices which outline ways of speaking about emotions and of acting out and upon bodily feelings within everyday life' (Burkitt 1997, 43) I am suggesting that the counselling session is a place where the social subjectivity of the social actor within that context is named through real or imagined 'feeling' and is then reflexively assigned meaning via socially organized emotion words and concepts. Counselling is useful as a backdrop because it acts as a micro structure of socio-emotional life. Within this interactional context, a 'structure of communication' is enacted between therapist and client, where feelings and emotions are negotiated in relation to self and other. It is an ongoing reflexive process. If we take the counselling session as a set of meaningful actions or 'overlapping frames' (Goffman 1974) then each frame incorporates much more than the stated activity. For example, the way language and language like signs are communicated, the way paralinguistic cues are assembled (e.g. facial expression) all reflect the transmission of information that gradually takes place within the session – until the signs mean to the sender what they mean to the recipient. This way of co-ordinating and co-orienting leaves all sorts of meanings transmitted through gestures and small talk which is routine to the session and indicates not only the meanings being transmitted but, more importantly, the formation of these meanings within a given culture or society. Emotion is central to the meaning formation of the session and to understand the meaning of emotion words is about our ability to envisage a 'complicated scenario' (Lutz 1998) that involves far more than bodily 'feeling' – it means incorporating moral viewpoints, personal and social goals, whole sequences of events – it means understanding the cultural signs and symbols of particular contexts and the social actor making choices about naming, via emotion words and concepts, how he or she 'feels' in relation to cultural meanings. The constitution of emotion is embedded within social meanings, reflecting social mores rather than named internal, organic states alone, while feeling is a real or imagined property of the living, breathing body that literally connects the body of the social actor to the social body through the naming of real or imagined bodily sensations or 'feeling' as emotion words and/or concepts. This basically means that bodily sensations or 'feeling' is used as a barometer of social values, goals and personal views while meanings for emotion are reflexively introduced to name feeling states and feelings states are used to reify emotion words – thus constructing an emotional habitus. Overall, counselling may be seen as one place that incorporates a variety of shared cultural meanings, boundaries and constraints that anchor both client and therapist into reality by 'definite, precise and surprisingly universal social mechanisms' (Goffman 1974) which are constantly organizing the situation for the social actors. The way the individual expresses thinking and feeling is not the product of the internal subjective state alone, but a mirror of the social world encapsulated in the room and informs the therapist therefore not only about social subjectivity but also a subjective sociality. Thus, the project of therapy illustrated by 'the session', extends far beyond the consulting room and in fact reflects how therapist and client inhabit their psycho-social world and the construction of their 'emotional habitus'.

The emotional habitus is the site where emotion and feeling, representing socialized objectivity and subjectivity, are brought together in an ongoing reflexive process which is highly dependent upon social meanings. This is shown in the research I introduce which found that emotions used to describe feelings were also influenced by the sex and gender identity categories of the social actors involved. This is quite revealing because it is often assumed that emotions are essential or biological components of self and therefore 'fixed' in their meaning. However, my research (Moon 2002, 2009) with 70 therapists over the past decade, indicates that the naming of emotion for feelings is influenced by the social meanings inherent within society for gender, sex and sexuality while the decision to identify as male or female, man or woman, lesbian, gay or heterosexual appears to be influenced as much by the way sexual feelings are named in relation to socially organized meanings for self and other. This was further illustrated when therapists stated that through the benevolence of 'age' and 'experience' they no longer wanted to isolate sexual feelings inside a specific identity category because this felt limiting. In fact, they seemed more open to reflection and to the challenges of reflexivity and stated their naming of 'felt' experiences moved beyond the meanings encapsulated in traditional categories for gender and sexuality. This was rather remarkable and I discovered that those interviewees who were familiar with queer theory and even named themselves as 'queer' were more likely to interrogate the links between feeling and 'identity' categories, while feeling and emotion appeared central to the construction of personhood. As Valentine (2006, 248) concludes, 'identity categories disable certain kinds of desires being validated' and therefore 'talking about desire' in 'the form of its expression through speech' not only allows us to understand 'the politics' of categorizing 'sexual' and 'gendered' experiences (p. 248) but also enables us to understand how sexual feelings or what may be referred to as 'erotic desires' may be expressed in ways that cannot be accounted for by identity categories.

Finally, I suggest in this chapter how queer communities offer an alternative and more liberating way of freeing the body and its concomitant feelings from the rigidity of emotion and the way it has been used to satisfy a heteronormative agenda. As a radical perspective, and through the use of queer theory, I explore an emerging queer praxis, what this means and the way this may be used to shift meanings when working with queer and non-queer clients in a 'communicative, interpretative and representational' context (Corber and Valocchi 2003). There is a push towards the liberation of feeling, a democratization of feeling that ultimately will allow for a queer praxis to emerge which is based upon what I refer to as 'poly-emotionality' – the ability to name feeling, especially sexual feelings, toward self and others, regardless of sex, sexuality and gender but dependent upon the context and its meaning at any given time. Using therapy as a site of contestation, I will introduce research to illustrate the way heteronormative discourses are given legitimacy within therapy. I then use the internal conversation, to highlight the way 'feeling' and emotion words and concepts, used to co-ordinate categories of sex, gender and sexuality, no longer fits with expected patterns. In fact, most therapists, regardless of sex, gender or sexuality are open to debating how sexual feelings are not confined by gender, sex or sexuality but by discourses, including therapeutic discourses, that limit the availability of debate in relation sex, sexuality, gender, emotion and feeling. They show how emotions and feeling are used to maintain the very categories they believe are no longer useful. These questions may be used to invigorate meanings embedded within therapeutic contexts.

The Research

As a social theory, the work of Pierre Bourdieu, in particular the writing on 'cultural field', 'habitus' and 'bodily hexis' may be usefully deployed to analyse the therapeutic context. It can contribute to a critical interrogation of the 'field' of therapy and the way it is formed, interpreted and how it is presented. Bourdieu refers to the 'partly unconscious' taking in of 'rules, values and dispositions' as 'the habitus'[3] which go on to produce the 'bodily hexis' where 'agent's bodies and bodily dispositions' reflect the habitus of values and imperatives (Webb et al. 2006, 36/37) of their different 'cultural fields'. Therapy is ripe for such an interrogation. The idea of 'field' is especially useful and therefore, before moving into the work of Bourdieu and what this may mean for therapeutic constructs, I want to introduce the research I have conducted over the past decade and in particular the research from my latest ESRC funded project. In doing this I am setting the background for the notion of field and habitus which will allow me to highlight how emotion and feeling are governed by the social.

---

3   Webb et al. (2002, xii) define the habitus as a concept 'that expresses', on the one hand, the way in which individuals 'become themselves' – develop attitudes and dispositions – and on the other hand, the ways in which those individuals engage in practices. An artistic habitus, for example, disposes the individual artist to certain activities and perspectives that express the culturally and historically constituted values of the artistic field.

The Study

The most recent ESRC[4] funded research conducted between October 2007 and
May 2009, was a nationwide study. It involved 40 therapists (10 gay male; 10
bisexual; 10 lesbian and 10 heterosexual) who were either Chartered (British
Psychological Society); Accredited (British Association for Counselling and
Psychotherapy) or Registered (United Kingdom Council for Psychotherapy)
which means they have at least 450 hours of theory and practice. Data taken from
episodic interviews lasting a minimum of one hour was analysed using grounded
theory and narrative analysis. This added to research with 30 qualified therapists
between 1999 and 2000 (Moon 2002) using one hour long semi structured
interviews and analysed using grounded theory. All therapists had experienced
their own therapy for at least 40 hours. Therapeutic models[5] named by therapists
from both studies involved a broad spectrum of those made available to the public
either privately or through voluntary sector/National Health Service centres. They
included: Cognitive Behavioural Therapy (CBT); Psychosynthesis; Transactional
Analysis; Neuro Linguistic Programming; Gestalt; Systemic; Psychodynamic;
Psychoanalytic; Jungian; Person Centred; Feminist; Integrative and Behavioural.
Demographically, all 70 therapists were aged from 28 to 70 years, able bodied
and predominantly white and middle class. They had been working as qualified
therapists for anything between three and 30 years. This is important to include
as most therapy training courses do not consider social demographics important
– an issue I will raise again later in the chapter. Although I worked to have
categories of an equal representation for heterosexual, lesbian, bisexual, and gay
male sexualities, and male/female sex and gender, the research was not adequately
inclusive of trans therapists or clients and I hope to extend this study in the future.
Also, in outlining the field of therapy, therapists reported how their experiences
in training did not reflect societal representation with virtually all interviewees
saying the bulk of their training cohort was white, middle-class, heterosexual, able
bodied and female in most training institutions at the time of their training between
seven and 20 years ago. Sex, gender and sexuality were rarely, if ever, addressed in

    4   I would like to thank the Economic and Social Research Fund (ESRC) for providing
a small grant to enable this research to be conducted at Warwick University who I would
also like to thank for their time, unending support and resources.
    5   The debate about models and approaches often fails to delineate what these mean.
My own understanding is taken from training where we were informed that there were three
main approaches (Interpretative, Humanistic and Cognitive-Behavioural). The transpersonal
was added later as a fourth approach. Within each of these approaches any number of
models may exist. This stance would prevent the limited outlook presently governing some
teaching e.g. the British Psychological Society dictates that practitioners must know at
least one 'model' in depth for Doctoral level study. A failure to understand more than one
model at this level is shown in the rapid rise of CBT. Knowledge of an 'approach' would
mean incorporating far more models and therefore offering clients a much wider access to
understanding their distress.

training. The professionalization of therapy, its ever increasing marketable value and its insurgency into public service settings (education, NHS, family, law) is beginning to alter this profile but there is still resistance to change.

Field and Habitus: The Impact on the Therapeutic Domain

Bourdieu (1977) introduced the concept of a 'cultural field' as a metaphor to explain how certain discourses and activities are produced and authorized via 'institutions, rules, conventions, categories, designations and appointments which constitutes an objective hierarchy' (Webb et al. 2006, x). The 'field' refers to 'the always existing, obligatory boundaries of experiential context' which 'engender and require certain responses, 'hailing' the individual to respond to themselves and their surrounding in specific ways to the point of habituation' while the habitus is 'the collective term for this array of dispositions' (Adams 2006, 514). The field of therapy involves 'habituating' people to the language and regulatory functions of therapy and this means structuring their knowledge so they take in rules, systems, laws, values and dispositions established by and through predominantly heteronormative meanings which give legitimacy to certain discourses presented as therapeutic models and approaches. These meanings are 'a part of us' as 'we are a part of them' and are taken into the session, acting as a backdrop to what takes place between therapist and client. Thus, as Adams (2006, 514) concludes, 'the field instantiates us as subjects and reproduces social distinctions via the enactment of habitus'.

The Field of Therapy

Although it may consider itself 'apolitical',[6] in fact therapy it is not a neutral field and is therefore 'already implicated in the production, dissemination and naturalization of repressive ideas and acts' thereby providing support for the very structures it purports to ignore (Webb et al. 2006). This operates primarily through language, either by ignoring the socio-political links of therapy to the social world, or by using the language of therapy to deny the validity of political meanings, rejecting political questions and instead locating meanings inside therapeutic concepts such as 'acceptance', 'defence mechanisms', 'cognitive distraction' thereby softening the blow of prejudice and refusing to tackle the insubordination of sex, sexuality and gender. Therapy represents how the social understanding of what constitutes mental health and mental illness i.e. the emotionality of the

---

6   Ironically, this is proving not to be the case. Despite counsellors and psychotherapists denying the politics of their profession, they are presently embroiled in a series of moves against the Government who wish to forcibly regulate therapy through the Health Professions Council.

general public, is embedded in the social and political ideals as represented through rules, institutions, conventions etc. and these are circulating within the therapeutic relationship reflexively forming its 'emotional habitus'. What we have witnessed over the past century is the way heterosexuality presides over these social functions so that a heteronormative structuring of what constitutes the everyday psychology of the general population has taken place to the point this is considered both 'natural' and necessary. For example, 'homosexuality' as a mental illness or form of personhood and identity was one of the 'dramatic social transformations that accompanied the rise of industrial capitalism and the emergence of the nation state' (Corber and Valocchi 2003, 2). Then, as now,[7] the push towards 'normalization' is the push towards a classed, racialized, able bodied, sexed, gendered and sexualized version of 'mental health'. Certainly my own research interviewing 70 therapists at different ends of the past decade has consistently shown this to be the case. The field of therapy is shown to be embedded within the values of heteronormativity, producing and reproducing discourses that maintain this social and emotional ordering. As shown earlier, all therapists I interviewed acknowledged that they had trained at institutions where heterosexuality was the normative structure, gender was primarily heterosexual female and most trainees were middle-class (by their definition) white and able bodied. Heteronormative discourses written into the training courses, included those around relationships, kinship structures and psychological structures such as the unconscious and psychodynamics. As Danielle[8] remarked:

> All models are in a heteronormative framework. Examples include the idea of the unconscious and the family ... All constellations are heterosexual ... No room for anything whatsoever as non-heterosexual ... the word "family" is used in a very heteronormative sense.

And Louisa, a lesbian therapist, added that therapy is out of step with 'the rest of society' because to those constructing the meaning of therapy 'normality's therapeutically healthy' adding:

> However, in the first place, they're ... they're not presenting an inclusive picture ... Like ... "Childhood and Lower Unconscious": *completely* heterosexist. *Nothing* about what's it like to be, um, a different child ... a different teenager: that for *me* ... I was *different*, you know.

---

7   As I speak, the South African runner Caster Semenya who won gold in the women's 800 metres race is under bodily interrogation for gender variation because it was deemed 'unnatural' that she won in the time presented. The debate is showing that Caster is in fact beyond the 'male/female' binary established and her 'body' does not conform to heteronormative fictions which are taken as established fact.

8   All names are pseudonyms.

Additionally, a very small number of therapists interviewed had trained in sex and/or relationship therapy and again, the overriding narrative is one that serves heterosexual assumptions. In effect, the lack of recognition awarded to anything other than heterosexuality is staggeringly obvious and goes without challenge. Thus, therapy, or rather those shaping the field of therapy, invokes a persuasive and political rhetoric that maintains not only heteronormativity but a heteronormative psyche. As Elena, a heterosexual therapist admitted, her training included couples therapy:

> It was, I mean there was a lot of emphasis on it, ... but primarily from a heterosexual viewpoint, but in terms of you know, what it is to be female, what is it to be male.

Likewise, in teaching sex therapy, hetero-sex is again taken as the norm. The body is framed within a heterodoxical structure, where, as Pietra stated:

> I mean the problem is always when there's something wrong with intercourse ... defined as penetration ... penis in vagina ... obviously ... And the assumption is that that's what clients want to do. Like successful penetration. ... It's also enshrined in the definitions of the problem and the solutions, the training programme ... yeh ... But, at the same time, you know, it still leaves in place what about heterosexual or bisexual women who may not be into penetration like, or heterosexual or bisexual men who might not be into penetrating.

Thus, people in positions of authority within the field of therapy maintain the values of heterosexuality as normative by refusing to recognize anything other than heterosexuality. They impose their own authoritarian meaning on the shaping of knowledge to such an extent that training now consists of its own discourses and style of language which 'determines what is seen ... what things are valued, what questions can be asked and what ideas can be thought' (Webb et al. 2006, 13). Although it would be unfair and incorrect to suggest that no lesbians, gay men or bisexual people are involved in teaching, it seemed to me from the research that they quite often tried to 'fit in' to the field of normative therapy. Often they had been students on the very same courses, had seen a gap in the teaching and then returned to offer a course on 'sexuality' or 'gender'. This rarely challenged heteronormativity, and was often embedded within normative understandings of relationships, family structures, childhood. Compromising rather than challenging. In effect, the lack of recognition for non-heterosexual sexualities extends to non-recognition of new structures permeating through non-heterosexual societies e.g. family structures challenged by polyamory and how this offers new insights into emotionality, relationship and sexual meanings. Thus, non-recognition allows for the domination of heteronormative values, rituals and rules 'which constitute an objective hierarchy, and which produce and authorize certain discourses and activities' (Webb, Schirato and Danaher 2006, 21). These become embedded inside the life story of the social actor where they constitute the 'inner dialogue' of beliefs, feelings, ideas and thoughts that are mediated via agency. For those who go 'into' therapy, revealing this inner dialogue is central to understanding whether or not feelings, thoughts, ideas and beliefs exhibit mental health or mental illness.

Silenced Voices and the Inner Dialogue – The Habitus

Embedded within, and emerging from, 'heteronormative' structures has emerged the social role of 'therapist' which although it may claim to be benign, is actually a politicized and political identity. The therapist as 'expert', far from offering individual freedom, is arguably constrained by the same normative structures that fail to recognize sex, gender and sexuality. Arguably, the therapist operates with a distance and separateness that works towards assimilation and a mental health economy based on heteronormativity. What this suggests and what was confirmed in my own research is that heterosexuality is 'naturalized' through conversations and 'talk' via therapeutic models that go on to reproduce a 'normative, taken for granted heterosexual world' (Kitzinger 2006, 187). An obvious example of this in therapy is shown in an earlier chapter by Ian Hodges who addresses the role of psychoanalysis and the way this particular discourse or social script underpins the logic of heterosexuality. Its strategies of gender coherence and sexual stability form a structure that is made apparent in maintaining heterosexuality – to the point where anything other than heterosexuality is marketed as abject 'failure'. Sex, sexuality and gender are usually divorced from the mainstream of therapy training courses and trainees are excluded from conversations, information or discussions that question the impact of these social forms on agency and/or the process of reflexivity. As one heterosexual therapist said to me, during her training, sex, sexuality and gender did not figure because, in her words:

> You are not a sexual being … You haven't got a libido. It's like we're talking about something in the middle of the room and we're trying to pretend it's not there …"I can't see it" … "I don't know what you're talking about". So it's not talked about, it's not looked at, there's no literature … We were not told to look at literature. We were not given any training on any of the University courses I attended.

The refusal to sanction discussion and debate about sex, sexuality and gender is a way of academically 'stonewalling' the meanings of non-heterosexuality within therapeutic discourse so that conversational exchange and reflexivity is not deployed. Rather than interrogating the relational self and organizing a narrative that can endure recognition of the non-heterosexed, non-heterogendered and/or non-heterosexual other, such narratives are rendered invisible. One must ask what is the purpose of such an act and try to unpack that which is made invisible. In effect, it highlights the contradictory nature of therapy – on the one hand attempting to commandeer a study of subjectivity, while on the other countenancing this with social and moral restraints towards sex, gender and sexuality.

In light of the above, interrogating the 'internal conversation' or 'silent speech' by asking therapists to talk about themselves and their thoughts and feelings towards lesbian, gay, bisexual and trans clients, that is, to be reflexive, offers one way of showing us what the social actor (e.g. therapist) understands about social and personal meanings for sex, genders, sexualities, emotion and feeling, their interrelationship and how/when/why/where related 'emotions' are imposed onto the feeling body. The research I have collected over the past decade (1999–2009) has consistently shown that the naming of emotion relies on the 'internal conversation' that operates within the session and leaves therapists naming the feelings of their client as well as their own feelings in response (Moon 2007). However, with no input on sex, genders or sexualities throughout training, it seems that therapists are limited in their understanding of feeling in relation to emotion and identity. Not only are therapeutic training courses embedded within heteronormative structures that represent certain value systems in relation to race, ethnicity, class, sex, sexuality and gender but, interestingly, all therapists recognized this trend. However, all felt unable to rigorously challenge it because, as they said, they are either excluded or discouraged from discussing, debating or divulging anything about sex, gender or sexuality throughout training, are rarely exposed to anything other than therapeutic models which present heterosexuality as normative while emotion is lodged firmly within 'the biological'. As Louisa stated, her role became difficult throughout training, because as she openly challenged normativity within the group she was left believing herself to be 'a nuisance', and 'an outsider':

> So I have to come in as challenger. And I mean really it's the *group* that I have the problem with ... because they felt I was al ... always questioning, always challenging; and this was a nuisance ... basically. You know, sit down, shut up and stop being useless – but not in those words, because they were too polite ...

while Jade a bisexual therapist, also felt the pressures:

> I mean this guy, this particular guy had made a cup in pottery for his counsellor and I was in the counselling room one day and his counsellor said he wanted a cup of tea but there wasn't a cup and he didn't like to use that cup because it had been made by this gay guy, and he didn't like to use that cup, and another counsellor, come in and said is there any cup and. I said well there is that one but its been made by so and so, and she said I don't like the vibe of that cup ...

Everyday practices are shaped by training, not just in relation to therapeutic practice but in relation to the way non-heterosexual trainees experienced their own acts and conversations monitored and altered by their training. Open transgression of heteronormativity led to various charges that led to trainees being aware of not fitting in, being excluded and in many cases, being completely isolated. Thus, the formation of the emotional habitus as a structuring as well as structured system, is also revealed for those who fail to subscribe to heteronormativity. In Bourdieu's language, the formation of the habitus matches the logic of the field through the unwritten 'rules of the game' or 'doxa' which are 'underlying the practices within that field (Maton 2008). It is a relational structuring of habitus and field where the individual gathers a 'feel for the game' so that 'you feel comfortable, at ease, like a "fish in water"' (Maton 2008, 57). However, for those who are outside of 'the game', it becomes obvious that they are left to struggle alone and although they can 'fit in' it is provided they internalize meanings framed via the dominant group. Feeling is used as a central component of the emotional habitus and, to a large extent, habitus is all about 'feeling' co-ordinated and co-oriented towards others in order that we feel we are all playing the same game! It is clear that the role of 'feeling' in relation to bodies, practices, field and habitus is beyond regulation and yet regulatory functions imposed through the field via emotion words and concepts, may inhibit feeling.

Therapists were quite aware of the way feeling was inhibited. Even more surprisingly, the therapists I interviewed believed that the present understanding of how sexual feelings are understood in relation to sexual identity within therapeutic training and texts did not fit with their own sexual and social experiences (Moon 2009). In fact, in these intimate conversations, it was shown how they are forming new relationships between field and habitus which appear to be about allowing themselves to assign new meanings to the feeling body in relation to sex, sexualities and genders. Quite often, therapists felt restricted by sexual and gender identity categories and shunned these 'fixtures' as emotionally and socially problematic. This fits with Valentine's earlier suggestion that we should move beyond identity categories to a more specific understanding of 'erotic desire' and I suggest, to a point where we explore the sexual habitus of people in order that we understand how feeling 'comfortable' or 'at ease' is related to the contextual field of gender and sexuality and is a socialized rather than natural concept. For example, during the interviews, it felt as though therapists were revealing, in some cases for the first time, their 'inner dialogue' (Archer 2003) that had remained hidden throughout training. For example, the following therapists who identify through present categories all revealed their feelings in relation to 'the other'. Dana, a heterosexual therapist, described herself as having: 'a very traditional identity. I am married to my husband and we have two children'. Later in the interview, in a discussion about feelings, gender and emotion, Dana admitted 'I'm 80 per cent heterosexual with a tiny piece of me that might be gay' and began to talk about her feelings towards another woman during her training as a therapist:

> It felt kind of romantic and it felt ... well, if things were different we might both..
> I think we both kind of knew but it was never said ... because I am married
> ... I had kind of wanted to act on it but I don't want to act on it ... but it felt
> wrong because I was with somebody and I don't want to hurt his feelings. As
> a heterosexual person ... yes, I see myself as being a wife. But not just a wife

either. I'm a person in my own right as well, but I think I notice the privileges still and the prejudices that are still there.

and Cecile, a lesbian therapist told me:

> I mean I'm thinking at the moment of a friend of mine who's a therapist who self defines as bisexual by inclination and lesbian by choice. Which I thought was quite an interesting way of defining it. I suppose in a way I could say the same about myself. I do find myself sexually attracted to certain men but uhh but I wouldn't ever choose now to have a relationship with a man after my past.

while Patricia, a heterosexual therapist in her mid-60s revealed:

> I did have a crush on my supervisor. I had ... I didn't realise it at the time but she actually came out to me as lesbian just as she was leaving and I was just devastated all round and I did actually feel a sexual attraction towards her, but that was the first time I felt a sexual attraction towards a woman, whether I am a late developer I do not know
>
> I: but what was the devastation
>
> P: she was leaving
>
> I: oh ok
>
> P: she was going ..., and I was so gobsmacked I couldn't say anything for the entire session, in fact she went to fetch me some reviving salts or something [laughter]
>
> I: did she know how you felt
>
> P: yes, well yes
>
> I: what did you like about her
>
> P: oh [laughter] she was warm and comfortable and large and an all enveloping hug and she was gentle and understanding and she had a nice soft bosom yeah, those sort of things
>
> I: Did it take you by surprise that you felt that you liked her?
>
> P: well, I don't know I can remember I suppose it did take me by surprise, I mean we are going back a few years we are going back what 10 years at least if not more, so I was having an adolescent crush on her at that point

I: do you think it was an adolescent crush, I mean if we go with the idea of the person then isn't it ok to feel that?

P: yes, but I can't imagine I can't imagine having sex with another woman other than hugging and cuddling, but I can't imagine doing that nude, and I can't imagine anything in the genital area that just doesn't do anything for me at all

I: does it have to be? is that what you would have to do?

P: I think I'm more aware of finding of the women attractive now and I mean I certainly have a sexual transference in my own therapy to the therapist and she doesn't know about it now [laughter], and its gone and you know it just happened for a while and it's gone

and Gerry, a gay male therapist stated:

I think I've always defined as a gay man. I think as I get older umm I'm more open to the possibilities and opportunities of relationships with women. Although at the moment I wouldn't say I'm in a space or a situation where I would have one. And maybe there's something about growing older as well. You know. As you do mature, as you do kind of umm get grips on, on what's going on internally then you have, then you have this freedom.

Thus, there is a dissonance between the inculcation of 'knowledge' and the narrated social and sexual experience of individual agents. Although throughout training, therapists bring into focus the relationship of their field-habitus, no doubt nurtured in relation to social structures and individual agency, this is always embedded within the social. However, it appears that the democratization of feeling operates through the freedom to allow a broader and more inclusive thinking and feeling – one that incorporates the body and the social, feeling and emotion, structure and agency. This raises two significant issues. First, the way formative knowledge is shaped about sex, genders and sexualities for and of 'feelings' as shown by the use of emotion words and concepts in everyday social life; and second, how silent speech about 'erotic desire' could, if made more transparent, circumvent discussion about identity and therefore fit with a queer understanding of selfhood and subjectivity.

Queer Praxis

Originally, LGBT populations formed a collaboration of thinking and feeling toward the oppressive 'heterosexuality' by awkwardly slotting alongside each other and collectively subscribing to the idea of an LGBT minority. The rise of minoritarian models led to the idea of LGBT identities whereby the heterosexual/

non-heterosexual binarism is brought into existence. In effect, 'the boundaries between homosexuality and heterosexuality were fixed and impermeable' (Corber and Valocchi 2003, 3). Out of this developed identity based politics. This has meant that LGBT therapeutic perspectives concentrate on, and advocate, identity based interventions. More recently, poststructuralists have argued that there is no such thing as a subject who is separate from, and prior to, social structures as 'the subject' is 'constituted in and through them and thus is neither autonomous nor unified but contingent and split. Subjectivity is not a property of the self but originates outside it and therefore is unstable' (Corber and Valocchi 2003, 3). However, this knowledge is not incorporated into therapeutic discourses where subjectivity is considered as a property of, and central to, the formation of self. In other words, all knowledge relating to sex, gender and sexuality is subordinate to the institutionalization of heteronormative ways of understanding 'the self' and selfhood.

In comparison, my research found that a number of interviewees were influenced by and through queer theory and designated a queer positionality. They referred to being 'queer', 'trans' or 'genderqueer', and had broken heteronormative meanings by applying queer theory to their everyday practices. For example, Maya commented how she assumed 'everyone' found men and women attractive because that was how she approached her queer world. Rather than locating this within a framework of pathology and thereby designating her desires to one gender, she acknowledges these feelings and in doing so, despite the interruption of traditional social mores, is free to unpack their meanings in relation to gender identification:

> I found men and women attractive. And then I think in my late teens two things … the X Files where I thought it's not Mulder or Scully it's Mulder and Scully so that dates me as well and secondly when my boyfriend at 6th form, I remember we were chatting in bed about stuff and he was like "Oh, so which girls would you fancy at school". And I was like "Oh brilliant question" so I told him. You know. And so "which boy's at school do you fancy then" and at that point he recoiled slightly and that point I was like "Oh, right okay. It's not equal".

And she continues to interrogate the meaning of her relationships and the meaning of gender and sexuality, stating:

> Something quite interesting happened about a month or two out of a relationship umm and I was thinking actually … the people I've been kind of crushing on recently have all been male/male identified. And I was chatting to a friend saying "Ohh I don't know where that leaves my queerness" and she was like "But you know, you're not stressing it's blokes you fancy. You're saying it's male or male identified". And that's quite a big difference. So you know, I think the queerness is still there.

The idea that sex, sexuality and gender are 'free floating' social representations for the body rather than fixed within the materiality of the body as an essential property begins to emerge. For Pietra, queerness captures a new formation of 'authenticity' in his queer identified body that allows for feelings to be freed from emotion as a signifier of the material body and he announces, in response to my questions about defining sexuality, that he defines as:

> ... an equal opportunities lover in a positive sense of the word. Fairly poly as well, although that keeps changing as well ... what that means ... moved from kind of ... over last 10, 13 years I've been in open relationships, umm closed relationships, promiscuous, abstinence, non-relationships. At the moment I guess in an open relationship which is fairly new though ... only 4 months or something ... so it's still early days. Wouldn't rule out having other, more prominent lovers within that ... but at the moment a kind of boyfriend, another gender queer, FT somewhere ... umm and yehh, casual sex ... mostly with kind of people I know.

This introduced new ways of interrogating sexuality and gender in relation to desire and rather than pathologizing his feelings, there was a freedom, a constant challenging of meanings, an ongoing reflexive purpose. As he stated when I asked how he explored these meanings:

> I've been exploring I guess ever since I started exploring ... I haven't really stopped. I've moved kind of from umm lesbian to bisexual to umm transboy to gender queer and kind of my preferences have changed over the years I guess in terms of the type of person I'm more open to umm I have been variously interested by kind of women, then kind of got curious about men again and then dated trans people for a while umm then kind of, kind of interested in non trans men for a while ... then started identifying as trans myself ... partly, partly in reaction to I guess, my sexual preferences myself because being with bioboyz and fancying them but not in heterosexual ways ... and kind of yehh I was meeting people that were attracted to my masculinity I guess and I started exploring it more.

And I follow up by asking him what it means emotionally, how he 'feels' and how he names these feelings. For Pietra, it simply means no longer using a 'pathologizing framework' or labelling what he is doing as 'bad' because it discriminates against non-normative understandings of sex, gender and sexualities:

> ... at the moment more than ever before I feel that I have sex with people who kind of ... who are interested in me, rather than some weird projection that I don't identify with or who are also open to, to shifts and changes within my you know, incongruities or you know, becomings within my gender presentation or within my sexuality as well. And obviously they have their own preferences of

their own ... like the person I'm seeing at the moment is kind of into trans boys but you know, at the same he's open to all kinds of other people and umm and is curious about, you know, where I'm gonna go next I guess. That's quite a good place to be. I mean it's scary in terms of like discrimination and all these things but it's exciting and it feels very authentic.

As the interviews progressed it became obvious that a number of people interviewed were transgressing normative and restrictive meanings for their way of relating to self and other through a queer theory discourse. It was noted how, within therapeutic discourses, these more recent and contemporary discourses are omitted and, as previously discovered, therapists rarely seem to have opportunities to deliberate what these may mean for constructions of personhood. In fact, far from being encouraged to assimilate these discourses into training, they are discarded and, as interviewees revealed, they become targeted as 'problematic' and representative of dangerous or 'taboo' discourses. Of course, if this were to be done it would surely mean that heterosexuality and heteronormative practices would tumble. As Pietra noted, at present we who are non-heterosexual in our everyday practices are tolerating the way heteronormativity penetrates the body and its meanings.

Conclusion

The influence of queer theory as a way of democratizing feeling and freeing it from the definition of emotion words and concepts, is essential if we are to liberate everyday sexual and gender practices to such an extent they introduce a queer praxis. The 'democratic imaginary' (Lewis 2008, 74) is essential if therapy is to be 'freed' from its own deeply embedded limitations. Queer theory may provide such a challenge, offering collective shifts in the way feelings and emotion are used to maintain binaries and dualistic thinking. Theoretically and practically, the world of therapy is hampered by compulsory heteronormativity. It fails to take issue with new meanings for sex, sexuality and gender and therefore fails to recognize, for whatever reason, the growing numbers of people who transgress heteronormative sexual and gender practices. While texts such as ICD and DSM represent the 'disorder' of sex and gender, queers are embracing disorder and constituting an approach that challenges 'the matter-of courseness of heterosexuality' that 'lies at the core of its cultural dominance' (Rosenberg 2008, 10). Taking issue with compulsion, queer repels the oppressive nature of identity categories and usurps their structural oppression. In comparison, therapy disguises normativity with the suggestion of seeking authenticity – an authenticity embedded within heteronormative practices. The meaning of personhood and authenticity within therapy means, I suggest, sitting with feelings (sometimes named discomfort, anger, hatred, disgust) towards non-normative accounts of sex, sexuality and gender and pinpointing how these have been socially ordered and imposed by therapists and therapy onto the non-heterosexual body. It means moving away from typical identity categories and accepting these as problematic – non-heterosexual sexualities and genders are not 'the same as' heterosexuality just as identifying as heterosexual is not 'the same' as intersexual, and identifying as lesbian is not the same as transgender – thereby rendering these identity categories as representations rather than biological projects. Feelings are products of a biological body simply because it is living, breathing, feeling and sensing. This is not the same as socially ordered emotions which are words and concepts shaped by societies, naturalized and embedded within everyday social narratives to describe 'feeling' in relation to social practices. Queerying these meanings will propel the democratization of feeling into the forefront and allow for a poly-emotionality to operate where emotions are no longer fixed to sex, gender or sexuality but are freely used to denote the variation in the materiality of the body. In this way, a new approach towards emotionality will emerge which will mean assigning emotion words and concepts to bodies no longer restrained by sex, sexuality and gender. It will mean no longer thinking in terms of rigid categories and corresponding how we feel towards the many forms of genders, sex and sexualities inscribed upon the body. For therapy, it means taking the opportunity to discuss and debate, without fear of reprisal, what our feelings mean, how they are named and what this naming may mean for personhood and authenticity.

References

Adams, M. (2006) 'Hybridizing habitus and reflexivity: Towards an understanding of contemporary identity', *Sociology* 40(3), 511–528.

American Psychiatric Association (1994) *Diagnostic and Statistical Manual of Mental Disorders*, 4th Edition (DSM-1V) (Washington, DC: American Psychiatric Association).

Archer, M. (2003) *Structure, Agency and the Internal Conversation* (Cambridge: Cambridge University Press).

Blumer, H. (1969) *Symbolic Interactionism: Perspective and Method* (London: University of California Press).

Bourdieu, P. (1977) [1972] *Outline of a Theory of Practice*, R. Nice (trans) (Cambridge: Cambridge University Press).

Burkitt, I. (1997) 'Social Relations and Emotions', *Sociology* 31(1), 37–55.

Corber, R.J. and Valocchi, S. (2003) *Queer Studies: An Interdisciplinary Approach* (Oxford: Blackwell Publishing).

Goffman, E. (1974) *Frame Analysis: An Essay in the Organisation of Experience* (Cambridge, MA: Harvard University Press).

Kitzinger, C. (2006) [2005] '"Speaking as a heterosexual": (How) does sexuality matter for talk-in-interaction', in D. Cameron and D. Kulick (eds), *The Language and Sexuality Reader* (London: Routledge).

Lewis, B. (2008) 'Democracy in psychiatry: Or why psychiatry needs a new constitution', in C.I. Cohen and S. Timimi (eds), *Liberatory Psychiatry* (Cambridge: Cambridge University Press).

Lutz, C.A. (1998) *Unnatural Emotions: Everyday Sentiments on a Micronesian Atoll and their Challenges to Western Theory* (London: University of Chicago Press).

Marshall, G. (ed.) (1994) *The Concise Oxford Dictionary of Sociology* (Oxford: Oxford University Press).

Maton, K. (2008) 'Habitus', in M. Grenfell (ed.), *Pierre Bourdieu: Key Concepts* (Trowbridge: Acumen).

Moon, L.T. (2002) 'The heterosexualisation of emotion: A case study in counselling lesbian, gay male, bisexual and trans clients', Essex University: Unpublished PhD thesis.

Moon, L.T. (2007) 'The heterosexualisation of emotion', in L.T. Moon (ed.), *Feeling Queer or Queer Feelings: Radical Approaches to Counselling Sex, Genders and Sexualities* (London: Routledge).

Moon, L.T. (2009) 'A psychosocial approach to counselling bisexual clients', ESRC funded research: Unpublished.

Rosenberg, T. (2008) 'Locally queer: A note on the feminist geneology of queer theory', *Graduate Journal of Social Science* 5(2).

Valentine, D. (2006) [2003] '"I went to bed with my own kind once": The erasure of desire in the name of identity', in D. Cameron and D. Kulick (eds), *The Language and Sexuality Reader* (London: Routledge).

Internet Resources

<en.wikipedia.org/wiki/caster_semenya>.

PART II
Relations of Resistance and Contestation

Chapter 5

Heteronormativity and Queer Youth Resistance: Reversing the Discourse

Julie Tilsen and David Nylund[1]

Twelve years ago, my (JT) partner Lauri and I were volunteering at the local queer youth drop-in center. It was dance night, and youth between the ages of 14 and 20 were filing in fashionably late. There was a mix of young men and young women and a few trannys as well. Most of the youth were white and there were a few African-American, Asian, and mixed-race youth as well, reflecting the dominant racial make-up of this northern US urban center. As we settled into our role as an 'adult presence,' we chatted-up some of the youth, checking in with those we knew from previous center events or other venues, meeting the latest main squeezes, introducing ourselves and the space to new comers, and getting up-close introductions to self-administered piercings and other-administered hickies.

One of the youth we knew from the center's softball team that we coached, introduced us to some members of her crew that were new to town. 'Huh,' the baby dyke mused, 'You guys don't look gay. Who's the butch and who's the femme?'

Introduction

What does it mean to 'look gay'? Did this young person believe that 'butch and femme' were compulsory roles to fill, requisite for looking properly gay, and that they were exclusive to other possible identities? What are the discourses that influenced these questions? What does it mean when gender identity specifications come from within the 'community,' rather than from the dominant culture. While my partner and I were being policed by people from the generation behind us, we have been left to wonder what impact our generation—that which

---

1   Authors' note: As a queer practice of accountability and to avoid taking up expert positions of speaking about a cultural group to which we don't belong, we intentionally sought the consultation of queer youth to inform and shape this chapter. We gratefully acknowledge the thoughtful and incisive contributions to this chapter, our work, and our lives made by Sarah Dack, Bren Dixon, Renu Kanda, and Courtney Slobojian.

came up and out during the Stonewall era—has had on the identity construction of young queers that have followed.

In this chapter we will address these questions by situating them historically within dominant discourses that continue, to this day, to influence our ideas about identity, sexuality, and gender. Our discussion will be organized around the question, 'how has the institutionalization—the cultural acceptance—of a "gay identity" reproduced some of the very oppressive limitations gay liberation originally fought against, particularly for contemporary queer youth?' The concept of homonormativity will be examined as a result of neo-liberal and assimilationist identity politics that maintain regulating effects on contemporary queer youth. Finally, we will discuss discursive therapy practices informed by post-structuralist and queer theories as a way to deconstruct such specifications for therapists who do not want to reproduce narrow, essentializing, and policing practices and that are founded on an ethic of justice, accountability, and solidarity.

The Birth of Homonormativity: Reverse Discourse Gone Wild

Bren is a 24-year-old Canadian queer white male. Bren explained that his way of showing up in the world failed to meet the standard gay male contingency. Not fitting into any of the typical categories that people seemed to want to put him (e.g., twink or bear), Bren took inventory of his appearance: He's too lean (not a gym queen); too pale (not at the beach or in the tanning booth); he has longish, curly, red hair (not preened enough); he wears comfortably worn clothes with a counter-culture vibe (he's not consumer enough); much of his body is covered in ink (he's not upstanding enough); and he's 'politically far-left' (he's not neo-liberal enough). For Bren, the trouble came mostly from gay men. 'I've been told to "get the hell out" of the bar because I'm not gay enough … I only go to the bar on ladies night with my women friends. It's the only time I can go somewhere and there's zero pressure on me.'

Courtney, a 25-year-old queer Canadian white woman concurs. Expressing her surprise at the amount of effort she has had to expend dealing with the policing effects from the queer community (she expected to deal with assumptions and judgment from the straight world), she states, 'this whole thing was constructed about me, for me' by other queers articulating specifications on issues from gender expression—'I was made into a femme dyke'—to choice of sexual partners: 'I told a friend that I had a crush on a certain girl and she said, "But is she even queer?" and I'm like, "Did you just ask me that question?" I think the term "queer" now has its own specific meanings.'

History and Discourse: 'Coming out' in Context

Most clinicians, like most of the general public, are not likely to be aware of the recency of the category 'homosexual'[2] and the subsequent markers, 'gay,' 'lesbian,' 'bisexual,' and 'transgender.' While people across time and place have engaged in a variety of sexual activities with various partners, including those of the same sex, never before had a category—*an identity*—been articulated to organize individuals based on their choice of sexual partners. The invention of the homosexual also required the invention of the heterosexual to stand against it. This obfuscation of history and the social construction of sexual identity serves to reify the notion of stable, natural gender and sexual identities and fuel the argument that people are 'born gay' while maintaining limiting binary notions of male/female and hetero/homo. The naturalizing of these specifications (for example, blue for boys, pink for girls; men are rational, women emotional; females are born with vaginas and clitorises and males are born with testes and penises) occurs through discourse and language.

Heteronormativity, the institutionalized assumption that everyone is heterosexual and that heterosexuality is inherently superior and preferable to any orientations outside of heterosexuality reflects the hegemonic effects of these discourses and the neglect of history. Homophobia, bi-phobia, and trans-phobia all stem from and are supported by heterosexism, which is then enforced by a gender binary system. It was heteronormativity, and its often violent, marginalizing, and humiliating tactics, that resulted in the Stonewall riots of 1969, the proud identification with a gay identity, and the subsequent demand for equal rights in all spheres of contemporary society, not to mention basic human rights of dignity and safety. By engaging in the practice of reverse discourse[3] gay activists carved out a place in society by 'being' the very thing that they were oppressed for.

What happens when a reverse discourse is hugely successful? Cultural theorist Lisa Duggan (2002) suggests that in the case of gay rights, homonormativity is one result of embracing an originally oppressive discourse all the way to your own place at the larger societal table. Duggan defines homonormativity as, 'a politics that does not contest dominant heteronormative assumptions and institutions but upholds and sustains them while promising the possibility of a demobilized gay constituency and a privatized, depoliticized gay culture anchored in domesticity

---

2 Foucault (1980) dates the invention of the term and category 'homosexual' to 1870. In part, this invention represented modernity's embrace of the scientific, a move from *ars erotica* to *scientia sexualis*. Foucault asserts that it points to not only the medicalization of sexuality, but the policing of it as well.

3 As a medium for the flow of power, discourse can be reversed by changing the direction of power without changing the foundational ideas on which the discourse relies (Foucault 1980). In this example, embracing an identity based on sexual partners and practices and developing a pedagogy of liberation based on it, serves not to overturn the discourse, but rather to change the meaning and value placed on it.

and consumption' (p. 179). By abandoning the radical and destabilizing purpose of the original gay rights battle (troubling gender norms and promoting what Rubin [1984] named sex positivity), homonormative queers have settled into a fairly bourgeoisie lifestyle—at the expense of those with less age, race, or class privileges or for those whom the this life does not fit.

The standard stonewall era 'coming out' narrative and its concomitant demand to be marked linguistically (i.e., identifying as 'gay' or 'lesbian,' 'twink' or 'dyke') limits peoples' capacity to maintain custody of their own story. As Bren and Courtney experienced, unique identity narratives are apprehended by a universal, pre-scripted text anchored in identity politics forged out of the life and death fight that was pre-stonewall survival. Consequently, specifications that instruct people on how to be gay and police them when they attempt to color their lives outside of the pre-inked lines are numerous. Hence, what once was, in a pre-stonewall context, liberating, transgressive, and resistant of heterosexual hegemony, has now become restrictive, normative, and compliant by reifying traditional notions of identity and family and embracing neo-liberal capitalist values. Where the claim of a stable gay identity ('I always knew I was gay') served to legitimize gayness in the show-me state of modernity (as well as during the current craze of privileging genetics and other medicalized constructions of identity), ushering in political access, social visibility, and cultural currency, these very hard-fought gains now function in delimiting ways, illustrating with great clarity the productive capacity of language.

Queer Theory: Honorable Resistance

Sarah is a 22-year-old white Canadian queer woman. She dated 'a queer man' for five years. 'We were constantly fighting against people telling us we were going to get married and have babies, that I'd quit school and have him take care of me. I was always fighting with my group of friends, fighting to make myself visible as queer. Like cutting my hair off—You had to go to some end of extreme of what queer means to make yourself visible within a circle of queer people if you're with a man.' After she ended this relationship, she found that she still had to fight to be seen on her own terms. 'I was out for dinner with my friend Kelly and we ran into someone we both knew. She asked if Kelly and I were dating and we're like, "no!" She asked "what are you?" Kelly said, "I'm a dyke" and I said, "I'm queer." She was like, "what!? Are you bisexual? Trisexual? What ARE you? What ARE you?" I decided that wasn't an appropriate question because it was meant to make her comfortable, not understand me how I want to be understood.'

Renu is a 26-year-old, first-generation Canadian queer woman from a traditional Indian family. 'I had trouble being labelled for the longest time. Queer is more an all-encompassing word. I take the stance you like who you like; you're attracted to who you're attracted to regardless of anything else. So queer, I say, is strange, odd, weird 'cuz it's kinda different. Queer is just one of those, it actually makes people think about what it is you're saying you are choosing to identify as. Like, if I say, "he's pretty hot" people say, "what! You're a big lesbo!" And I'm like, I didn't tell you that, did you just tell me that? Or they're like, "so you're bisexual." Where did that come from? Why are you choosing to ask me this? I'm Renu. Queer, strange, odd, weird. I'm a little different than what you might think.'

Overview

Queer theory is premised on the post-structuralist notion of non-essentialized identities. Gender and 'sexual orientation,' for example, are not viewed as naturalized or fixed characteristics located ahistorically and non-contextutally within individuals. Rather, these markers of social location are seen as fluid, contextually determined, socially constructed variables that shift and change in different contexts and at different times (Butler 1990). As a critical practice, queer theory interrogates the relationship between sex, gender, and sexual desire, situating these constructs within larger socio-cultural contexts including the intersection of such markers as class and race and the influence of consumer capitalism (Butler 1990; Foucault 1980; Halberstam 2005; Sedgwick 1990).

The intention is to complicate hegemonic assumptions about the continuities between anatomical sex, gender identity, sexual identity, sexual object choice, and sexual practice. As a critical practice, queer theory rejects biological theories of sexual identity and questions the usefulness of sexual and gender categories. Queer theorists ask: Who do these categories serve?

- Who do these categories include and whom do they exclude?
- Who has the power to define the categories?
- How are the categories policed?
- How do these categories change over time and across cultures? (Doty 1993).

As therapists and teachers of therapists-in-training, we find that these questions help us destabilize the truth status typically afforded the theories and models purveyed by and for clinical practice. (For more about this interrogation of clinical theories and practices see, Nylund and Tilsen 2006.) Further, queer theory invites us to be keenly aware of history, particularly the history of sexuality. In *The History of Sexuality,* Foucault (1980) asserts: 'No longer simply someone who participates in certain sexual acts, the homosexual begins to be defined fundamentally in terms of those very acts' (p. 101).

Queer Theory, Queer Therapy

How does queer theory influence our practice? As family therapists, queer theory supports our commitment to a practice that considers multiple levels of context and history. By rejecting the limits of binary-based, essentialized identity conclusions, we are provided a measure of conceptual freedom from the hegemonic assumptions of traditional theories of psychotherapy that reflect modernist constructions of identity. For example, well-meaning therapists, queer and straight alike, have traditionally been trained to encourage clients to 'come out.' This perspective has viewed clients that don't come out as having 'internalized homophobia' or of being 'in denial' of their 'authentic' self. From a queer theory perspective, this practice is problematic for several reasons.

First, the idea of internalized homophobia perpetuates the injustice of privatizing socio-cultural problems, in this case, homophobia and heterosexism. We utilize the narrative therapy practice of externalizing (White and Epston 1990) to locate problems more properly in their cultural context. This is a more socially just practice that affords people discursive space to consider their relationship to problems and their potential to act in resistance to them.

Secondly, the notion of a 'true' or 'authentic' self is premised on Western modern constructions of stable and essentialized identities that are independent of the world around them. Queer theory rejects such universal constitutions as deterministic, ahistorical and acontextual. Notions of authenticity erase the possibility of unique identity conclusions not necessarily marked by conventional language.

Furthermore, while claiming a sexual identity can provide a very powerful option for persons who identify as gay, lesbian, bisexual, and/or transgender, 'coming out' can also be another standard for sexual expression that people may feel obligated to meet. In addition, privileging the coming-out narrative can unwittingly work in the service of the institutionalization of heterosexuality. Foucault (1980) suggests that claiming a fixed identity as homosexual may be personally liberating but unintentionally privileging of heterosexuality. Lastly, coming out or being out, is not an equal opportunity endeavour. Issues of intersectionality must be considered as queers from various social locations and cultural contexts will have differing consequences within their communities.

Taking up this position allows us to listen 'outside the box' of the unquestioned discourses from psychiatry/psychology, medicine, humanism, and even gay and lesbian developmental models that influence young people. Furthermore, rejection of essentialist notions of identity construction and the psychosocial theories that support them allows for illumination of issues of power and oppression inherent in a heterosexist society and regulated through therapy practices born out of heterocentric assumptions. As such, queering our practice is an act of social justice and accountability.

Lost for Words

Not all experiences are accounted for by language or the categories that serve as linguistic short-cuts (e.g., gay, lesbian, bisexual). The notion of 'queer' is itself a critique of identities rather than a new constitution of its own. As such, it causes much dialogical consternation in our Western, modernist, binary-based culture of certainty. Queer' represents for all those people for whom labels don't or won't.

As therapists, what then, do we do? Trafficking in a cultural economy based on language in a profession dependant on conversation, this dilemma presents for us an invitation to reposition ourselves discursively with our knowledge as well as with our clients. Knowing that language is productive and not simply descriptive and that identities are discursively produced rather than essentially and deterministically fixed, we choose guiding questions such as:

- How can we use language and discourse in ways that invite a proliferation of possible identity conclusions and performances rather than discourses that mandate and regulate identities?
- What discursive positioning will allow queer youth's individual identity claims and lived experiences to be legible as acts of resistance to delimiting discursive power relationships that demand stable, fixed, and binary identities?
- How can we structure safety and allow discursive space that allows queer youth to bring all of themselves to therapy?
- What do we need to stay mindful of and how can we account for therapy practices that are not in solidarity with queer youths' preferred ways of being?
- As family therapists committed to relational work, we also ask:

  - How can we position ourselves at the level of discourse in order to consider the effects of dominant discourses on important people (e.g., parents, family members, other support figures) in the youth's life?
  - What is the relationship between broader cultural narratives and the individual narratives of the people involved with the youth?

We argue for a position of radical doubt toward all universalized 'truths' and assumptions about identity construction. This requires careful deconstruction and meaning-making of clients' internalized and decontexualized understandings of themselves. Borrowing from Foucault (1980), we suggest that to construct the history (and possible trajectory) of someone's identity construction it is imperative to do so through the lens of discourse and history. Because we situate our understanding of queer identity construction and 'coming out' within this historical discourse—which includes the history of sexuality becoming medicalized and regulated by psychotherapists—we experience queer youths' intentional rejection of fixed identities and their embrace of fluidity as an honorable act of resistance. In short, where others see pathology ('internalized homophobia' and/or adolescent 'defiance') we revel in their political activism.

As an example, the following vignette demonstrates how we apply queer theory to therapy practice.

Queering Therapy

Lesbian? Trans? ... Queer.

Angelica,[4] a Black Jamaican 17-year-old, came to see me (DN) at the local LGBTQ Counselling Center for assessment to determine readiness for hormone therapy. Accompanying Angelica was her stepmother, Brooke, a 52-year-old white women, who was supportive of Angelica transitioning from male to female. Angelica was very bright and engaging. She explained that she had been living full-time as a female for over a year. As I explored Angelica's story, she shared that she 'was not home in her body ... I knew something was different since I was 4 years old.' As she came into her teen years, Angelica thought of her different-ness as gay because she was attracted to young men. As a 14-year-old, the term 'transgender' was not something she was aware of and gender variance was rarely discussed or portrayed in popular culture or societal institutions. However, gay and lesbian representations were widely available to Angelica.

As our first interview continued, Angelica stated that gay identity did not quite fit for her. She said there was something, 'not right, missing' when she tried on those ideas. While attending the Gay/Straight alliance group at her high school, the staff advisor wondered if Angelica was transgender. The advisor's speculation made complete sense to her. Angelica recalled that day during our meeting. 'I thought, "that's it! I'm not gay, I'm transgender!"' Angelica felt empowered and found courage to begin living her life as a woman, both in private and public. In medical discourse, and among members of trans community, this is known as, 'real life experience' (RLE).

Coming out as trans to her family wasn't only a challenge for Angelica. Brooke reported her own period of transition and struggle while adjusting to the permanence of Angelica's transition. 'I wondered for some time,' Brook said, 'if it was just a phase. And I had just gotten used to her being gay, now this!' Brooke also had significant concerns for Angelica's safety. With time, she was encouraging of her stepdaughter's gender identity. A pivotal moment occurred, Angelica and Brooke shared, when they went shopping together for dresses and make-up. This proved to be a transformative and bonding experience for both women. Although Angelica's father was somewhat ill at ease with her transgender identity, he did attend our second interview. Because she was under 18 years old, Angelica needed parental consent to get hormone treatment and her father agreed to provide this according to the Harry Benjamin Standards of Care, the consensus opinion for medical and psychological care of transgender individuals (Butler 2004). Angelica qualified for hormone treatment. The Harry Benjamin standards state that people need to have three months of RLE and/or three months of counselling before qualifying for medical interventions.

Working within the pathologizing and medicalized system that provides the hormonal and surgical options that many trans people (such as Angelica) seek

4   Angelica has given her permission to have her story told in this format.

creates an ethical dilemma for us. Positioning ourselves within the politics of queer theory, we reject the universalized and expert constructions of gender, sexuality, and, more broadly, 'normal' that define this system. Trafficking in diagnostic categorizations such as so-called 'Gender Identity Disorder' has invited us to work through the dilemma by assuming a position of strategic essentialism (Spivak 1987). Until other structures and discourses are in place, GID is a strategic means for transgender clients to gain access to trans-friendly doctors and Sex Reassignment Surgery (SRS). Hence, we use the medical category of GID against itself to empower trans clients. Furthermore, as a way of challenging the opaqueness of the medical hegemony, we share our critique of GID. We believe that this transparency serves to honor and make room for individual client stories.

In therapy, Angelica would converse about her experiences in a trans youth group she had been attending. She focused a great deal on her feelings of not measuring up to the group members' ideas of passing. Angelica began to see how the group, while empowering on one level, was disciplining due to specifications of what it meant to be an 'appropriate' trans female. Angelica and I were unpacking the politics of gender by questioning the effects of homonormativity and more specifically, what we have come to call *transnormativity*. Critical, deconstructive questioning that problematizes binary constructions of gender and universal notions of identity is a cornerstone of queer theory. Through this process of inquiry, Angelica and I exposed the specifying discourses that had her measuring herself against transnormative standards that did not support her preferred way of performing her gender identity. One of the limiting criteria imposed by the group involved judgments surrounding Angelica's sexual object choice. The accusation that Angelica was not 'normal' emerged after she shared that, as her transition advanced, her sexual object choice changed from male to female. Angelica left the group thinking that there was something 'wrong' with her.

Queer theory challenges this kind of privatizing and pathologizing discourse that obfuscates broader cultural narratives (e.g., the gender binary, specifications for femininity, etc.) that influence individual narratives, in this case, that 'there is something wrong with me.' In response to this de-contextualized, self-incriminating comment, I asked her the following questions:

- Who gets to decide what is normal?
- Might these sexual and gender categories be more fluid than what is typically thought of?
- How did you fight off homophobia and trans-phobia to courageously honor your preferences and desires?
- What freedoms are possible if you stand outside of a gender and/or sexual binary system and fixed categories of identity?
- How might you inspire other queer youth to ward off the policing of gender and sexualities to live a life of their own preferences?

Furthermore, situating the group's understandings within the broader culture and acknowledging the effects of normative discourses on its members was critical, as well. This was important in order to subvert the reproduction of wrongly privatizing responsibility—casting blame—at the individual level. Angelica's liberation did not have to come at the expense of individual group members. By externalizing (White and Epston 1990) effects of normative discourses, Angelica was able to gain space for herself and the group members from these effects, thus inviting a contextualized understanding of and compassion for the group members. Angelica came into this understanding through questions such as:

- Do you think that trans people invented ideas of femininity and masculinity?
- How have other group members experienced gender policing?
- Have the gender police always been trans and queer people?
- What do you admire about some of the group members? What have some of them taught you that you want to carry forward in your own way?
- What are some possible differences in each individual's life that may influence them to more or less take up gender-typical presentations and practices?
- How can you honor peoples' personal preferences that may be different form your own without having to meet their criteria?
- Would you say that making room for a range of trans identities—including those that may be seen as gender-typical—helps to stand up to the policing?

These questions loosened the grip that homonormativity and transnormativity had on Angelica as we shifted the gaze from identitarian ways of living to the real effects of normative gender and sexuality that resides within the LGBT community. Engaged in a therapy informed by queer theory, Angelica reacted to these questions with deep thought and critical refection.

In our next meeting, Angelica said, 'I don't like the term trans as much anymore. It's too confining—queer fits me better.' This revelation led to another queer expansion for Angelica. She decided that, while continuing on hormones, she no longer desired sexual reassignment surgery. 'I don't need to have a vagina to be a woman,' she insightfully exclaimed. I was moved by her ideas of unhinging sex and gender from a narrow biological, medicalized view towards a more socially constructed version of sexuality and gender. Angelica's declaration of queer independence exemplifies the powerful utility and fruitful possibilities embedded within queer theory-informed therapy.

Conclusion … We've Only Just Begun …

Queer youth resistance to homonormativity can be viewed and leveraged through the lens of queer theory as a way to contextualize, historicize, and politicize the ever-changing landscape of youth identity development. As previously noted, while Foucault viewed the claiming of a gay identity as potentially liberating for individuals, he cautioned against its potential to reify heterosexuality as the norm. The great success of the modern gay rights movement that dates back some 40 years and the relative acceptance of gay identity (and the people associated with it) has led to the centering of a homonormative identity that has pushed to the margins those individuals embracing identities that don't define them neatly on the male/female, homo/hetero binaries. Bren, Courtney, Renu, Sarah, Angelica, and many others have in essence, returned to a Foucaultian sensibility, defining themselves not solely by sexual partners or gender expressions, but based on political values and ethical positioning that informs how they want to show up in the world. By reversing the successful reverse discourse that is contemporary gay identity, queer youth are re-working the meaning of sexual and gender identity in the post-stonewall landscape.

Although we find that queer theory offers a theoretical/political foundation that supports our preference for conceptualizations that oppose universal truth claims and the hegemony of the psychiatric system, in practice (and in life outside of the consulting room) we want to be sure that our theory—queer or not—does not take precedence over the lived experiences and preferences of our clients. Indeed, privileging clients' experiences over theoretical assumptions is a queer practice! While there has been a queer theory revolution in the academy that we can now bring into our applied work with individuals, families, and communities, we encourage clinicians and youth workers to stay close to the inspiring stories of revolution that are happening daily in the lives of youth such as Bren, Courtney, Renu, Sarah, and Angelica.

> Sit back and watch—watch this new generation unfold with new ways of being. You did things completely differently from how we're doing them because your context was so completely different … (Courtney)

References

Butler, J. (1990). *Gender Trouble: Feminism and the Subversion of Identity* (New York: Routledge).

Butler, J. (2004). *Undoing Gender* (New York. Routledge).

Doty, A. (1993). *Making Things Perfectly Queer: Interpreting Mass Culture.* (Minneapolis: University of Minnesota Press).

Duggan, L. (2002). *The Incredible Shrinking Public: Sexual Politics and the Decline of Democracy* (Boston: Beacon Press).

Foucault, M. (1980). *The History of Sexuality: An Introduction* (New York: Vintage).

Halberstam, J. (2005). *In a Queer Time and Place: Transgender Bodies, Subcultural Lives* (New York: New York University Press).

Nylund, D. and Tilsen, J. (2006). *Pedagogy and Praxis: Postmodern Spirit in the Classroom. Journal of Systemic Therapies* 25(4), 21–31.

Rubin, G. (1984). 'Thinking Sex: Notes for a Radical Theory of the Politics of Sexuality', in Carole S. Vance (ed.), *Pleasure and Danger: Exploring Female Sexuality* (Boston: Routledge & Kegan Paul), pp. 267–319.

Sedgwick, E.K. (1990). *Epistemology of the Closet* (Berkeley: University of California Press).

Spivak, G. 1987. *In Other Worlds: Essays in Cultural Politics* (Taylor and Francis).

White, M. and Epston, D. (1990). *Narrative Means to Therapeutic Ends* (New York: Norton).

Chapter 6

The Colour of Queer

Catherine Butler, Roshan das Nair and Sonya Thomas

Queer theory is often posited as being one of the world's newest academic disciplines, fit for the twenty-first century, with all the opportunities for embracing progressive, modern thinking. However, while queer theory presents as being all embracing, it has in truth been limited in its discussion of 'difference' to white middle-class norms, relegating non-white voices to the sidelines and footnotes of queer academic history. In negating non-white voices, and in failing to examine the impact of a white frame for queer theory, theorists have denied themselves and their students a rich and useful perspective. Patrick Johnson, a foremost, unique and rare black voice in queer literature, conjures up a culinary metaphor to capture this: 'While queer theory has opened up new possibilities for theorizing gender and sexuality, like a pot of gumbo cooked too quickly, it has failed to live up to its full critical potential by refusing to accommodate all the queer ingredients contained inside its theoretical pot' (Johnson, 2001, 18).

When race is discussed in queer theory, it can be done clumsily (Bergman, 1991; Moya, 1997; Ng, 1997). As one example, Gates (1999) suggests that 'contemporary homophobia is more virulent than contemporary racism' (p. 28), 'Mainstream religious figures – ranging from Catholic archbishops to Orthodox rabbis – continue to enjoin us to "hate the sin": it has been a long time since anyone respectable urged us to, as it were, hate the skin' (p. 29). However, statistics and statements such as these make no sense because the race (or gender) of the people attacked in homophobic violence is not reported. Fortunately, Gates (ibid.) goes on to urge us to consider that there is no 'measuring rod' (p. 29) of oppression upon which to measure different identities, and that such a rod would break when people hold multiple identities.

It is probably unfair to fault queer theory for its relatively poor oeuvre related to race and ethnicity because as a theory its anti-identitarianism is what makes it inclusive and transferable to multiple domains. However, it is *identity politics* that tend to bring the focus back to individual identities. As Ford (2007) rightly speculates, '(i)f gay identity is problematic and subject to a corrosive critique, mightn't other social identities be as well?' (p. 478), including race. However, Johnson and Henderson (2005) argue that for queer theory to ignore the range of multiple individual subjective positions it is not only 'theoretically and politically naïve, but also potentially dangerous' (p. 5). Indeed, Johnson (2005) asks what 'are the ethical and material implications of queer theory if its project is to dismantle all notions of identity and agency?' (p. 129). Cohen (2005), taking a different approach, suggests that queer theorists have established a dichotomy between heterosexuality and everything that falls outside of this. She critiques queer theory for neglecting to explore marginalization and privilege on the two sides of this generated dichotomy, rather than assuming that all queers are 'marginalized and invisible' and all heterosexuals 'dominant and controlling' (p. 25). Queer theory thus falls back into the familiar position it seeks to deconstruct, of 'powerful/powerless; oppressor/victim; enemy/comrade' (p. 45). This is the antithesis to queer politics' claim to interrupt dominant discourses and move beyond single-identity-based politics in recognizing multiple sites of oppression, and challenging prejudice and the agents that develop and sustain them. Therefore, for queer politics to be true to itself, it must reflect on its own complicity in (perhaps unwittingly) becoming yet another dominant discourse, with the power to subjugate others. The very idea of a queer self-identity can be construed as one that is only available to a minority of people within those who have same-gender desires/sex. This queer minority is often affiliated with those who are white, socially mobile, academic and predominantly Western (Bright, 1998). Therefore the term Queer needs to be used carefully, remaining mindful of who it represents and who has access to it.

And so, when it comes to the colour of queer, there is no glorious technicolour as we argue that queer remains framed in black and white. Most of the writing about sexuality and race comes from the humanities or in art (e.g. Gary Fisher, Joseph Beam, Marlon Riggs, Pratibha Parmar, Isaac Julien), rather than psychology. Indeed, the history of psychology/psychiatry's relationship with race and sexuality has been one of direct, and more recently, more subtle forms of oppression and pathologization. For example, the psychiatric diagnosis of 'drapetomania' once existed, which referred to the mental illness that would cause a slave to run away and whipping was suggested as treatment (Kutchins and Kirk, 1999). Today sees proportionally more black men represented in mental health wards and on psychotropic medication than their white counterparts (Bhui et al., 2003; Keating et al., 2000; Lloyd and Moodley, 1992). With regards to sexual minorities, homosexuality was considered a mental illness by the American Psychiatric Association until 1973, and by the World Health Organisation until 1992. Bartlett et al. (2009) report that in their survey of 1848 therapists in Britain, 17 per cent had attempted to help reduce or change their client's same-sex attraction. These facts demonstrate not only the historical, but also the contemporary subjugation that Black and Minority Ethnic (BME) individuals and sexual minorities experience.

In this chapter we will deconstruct practices of power that perpetuate discrimination, arguing that while queer theory does this for sexual identity, within this there is little discussion of racial identity. In the majority of writing about 'race', it is usual that it is BME issues that are discussed – thus assuming that white people do not have a race or that they are the norm against which 'the other' is to be compared. We will discuss blackness and whiteness as racial categories and consider their interaction with queer, charting their historical origins and exploring contemporary issues. We shall question the notion of a hierarchy of oppression and consider the use of language in queer communities. We hope this chapter will generate further debate and add to the value and range of existing literature.

Queering Colour

A Black and White Frame

Race is a social construction. Historically it was argued to be a biologically-based concept that was used to oppress and enslave non-whites. This happened in the seventeenth century with the racialization of slavery and the need for whites to justify their taking of power (Kincheloe, 1999). Since this time, white and black have been represented as opposites, as light/dark, angel/devil, good/bad (Haymes, 1996).

Who is Black?

The need to categorize and define who we are and where we fit in is an inevitable and largely invaluable element of our socialization. Much depends on who is doing the defining and assigning. The need to define and identify by colour historically has mattered only in terms of distinguishing and understanding what is 'not white'.

Skin colour has a long history of use as not only a mechanism of racially categorizing but also, consequently, of oppressing. The early nineteenth century saw the categorization of the three major races: Negroid, Caucasoid (or Europoid) and Mongoloid. Indeed, constructions of race were the very foundations of South Africa's system of apartheid, with pigmentation used to control access and rights throughout the political and judicial systems of the country. Floyd-James points out that 'we define no other ethnic population as we do blacks' (2001, xi) and that the word 'black' rapidly replaced 'negro' towards the end of the 1960s, when the black power movement in America had reached its peak. Therefore, to identify who is black and its corollary, who is therefore 'not white', remains for many essentially an exercise in attributing worth, with failings of character stereotypically attributed to complexions considered to be non-white; grounding along colour lines those who are considered powerful and those who are not.

Mason-John and Khambatta (1993) use the definition of black that was once used by the London Black Lesbian and Gay Centre as being those 'descended (through one or both parents) from Africa, Asia (i.e. the Middle East to China, including the Pacific nations) and Latin America, … the original inhabitants of Australasia, North America, and the islands of the Atlantic and Indian Ocean' (p. 9). This definition is wide and embracing and has proved useful to many therapists seeking to position themselves in relation to their clients' ethnic and cultural background.

While 'coloured' was once commonly used to describe people of African descent, 'people of colour' is now more widely accepted as a term that distinguishes those who are not white. However, it has also been criticized as suggesting that whites are not of a colour and therefore not considered in debates and discussions about race. It is interesting to note that the term 'coloured' has a different meaning amongst black Africans in some sub-Saharan countries. Here, it refers to someone who is neither black nor white – a mixed-race person. This term in such contexts is not considered a derogatory descriptor. Therefore one needs to be fully aware of the contexts in which such terms are used.

Black as a colour and an identity is, therefore, a relative construct. It can be homogenized to include everyone who is non-white or it can be fractioned amongst a group of non-white people to only include those who have a black heritage from Africa, to the exclusion of all other non-white people. Therefore, for a South Asian man, he can be black amidst white people, brown amongst black Afro-Caribbean people, and chocolate or 'wheatish'[1] amongst brown people, etc. Therefore, colour can only be understood as 'différance' (cf. Derrida, 1978). Derrida's idea of différance suggests that words and signs can only ever be approximations of meaning, and that true meaning can be gleaned by understanding the difference between these words from other words, and thereby meaning being always deferred.

It is interesting to note that in the UK, derogatory terms such as 'coconut' (brown on the outside but white inside) and 'banana' (yellow on the outside but white inside) are used to mark those African/Caribbean/South Asian and East Asian individuals respectively, who are deemed by others from their own ethnic background to have been corrupted by the West in their thoughts and actions and so 'act white'. The use of certain accents, dress, and even lesbian, gay, bisexual (LGB) sexuality labels and practices, can be seen as an appropriation of western ideology and culture at the expense of one's indigenousness. It also noteworthy that British South Asian youth may make conscious attempts to distance themselves from speaking Standard English, as this form of English is viewed (particularly when spoken by a non-white person) as a 'gay' marker (Jaspal, *personal communication*, 2009). Therefore, such groups adopt ghetto-speak or ebonics. However, racialized sign systems in gay-speak identify both the signifier and the signified. Therefore, it is not only the love-object that is racialized, but also their lovers. Culinary argots such as 'rice queen' (usually, an older white man who desires East Asian men), 'potato queen' (an East Asian man who desires white men), 'curry queen' (a white man who desires South Asian men), and 'sticky rice' (an Asian man who desires other Asian men) identify men on the basis of the race of the men they desire.

---

1   Hue also plays a major role amongst some brown (South Asian) people, with lighter ('wheatish') tones being considered the ideal. This ideal has created a major market for skin-whitening creams (e.g. 'Fair and Lovely') and has also been related to how beauty (particularly, female beauty) is constructed.

Who is White?

Just as there is no one way to be black, there is no one way to be white – this category includes a disparate group of ethnicities and nationalities that has expanded over time (e.g. in the US it was not until the nineteenth century that the Irish, Polish, Italians and Jews were considered white – Roediger, 2005). The concept of whiteness began following the Enlightment as colonialism and the slave trade associated whiteness with rationality, science, productivity, self-control and orderliness and those deemed non-white as primitive, lazy, irrational, violent and chaotic (Kincheloe, 1999). Whiteness is thus universalized and naturalized to become the unmarked, invisible, unquestioned and unexamined norm. White people are still taught to think of themselves as the average, the norm, morally neutral and the ideal (McIntosh, 1997).

Whiteness is thus not based on a common culture, language, history, religion, cuisine, philosophy or literature, but on a political arrangement of power and resources distributed by skin colour (Jay, 1997). However, whiteness also interacts with other areas of social difference: class, gender, sexuality – so that not all whites feel they have access to equal amounts of power (Kincheloe, 1999). Despite this, being a member of a group that also experiences discrimination (e.g. homophobia, disabilism, sexism, etc.) does not take away the benefits that come with white skin colour. When whites are taught about racism, they are taught about disadvantage for those from BME groups, however the corollary of this is not discussed – the advantages for white groups (McIntosh, 1997). Current thinking about racism is thus limited as it focuses on 'minorities' and oppression, and not privilege and advantage (Lucal, 1996). There are some universal white privileges, as McIntosh (1997) names in her now classic paper, for example:

- I see people of my race widely represented on the television and in newspapers.
- My children will be taught about people from their race at school.
- I can do well without being called a credit to my race.
- I can swear, dress scruffily, not answer mail without being seen as an example of the bad morals, poverty or illiteracy of my race.
- I will not be asked to speak for all people of my racial group.
- I can focus on racism without being seen as self-serving or self-interested.

Such privilege and qualities are transferred onto whiteness without being requested, as are fears and hostilities given a social history of racism and oppression (Jay, 1997). As Brod (1989) describes: 'privilege is not something I take and which I therefore have the option of not taking. It is something that society gives me, and unless I change the institutions which give it to me, they will continue to give it and I will continue to have it, however noble and egalitarian my intentions' (p. 280).

Since the civil rights movement, whiteness has been racialized – it is no longer taken for granted as the norm against which to assess and judge non-whites. White people are now in the position of having to find a language to talk about whiteness, to form a new white identity that is not divorced from the political historical oppression upon which continued white privilege is based. This is not with a false hope of erasing power differences and white privilege, but it is in the hope of creating open dialogue and opportunities for social change. Zetzer (2005) concurs that through open and honest multicultural dialogue we can begin to 'transform people and systems and turn intention into action' (p. 13).

A White Queer Theory

Whiteness is not queer when it is taken as the invisible norm. The examination of whiteness within queer communities is lacking. In the early 1990s, queer studies grew along parallel pedagogical and activist/campaigning lines (e.g. Queer Nation, ACT UP, lesbian avengers). Queer studies began by privileging one identity marker above all others, and so sexuality was explored at the expense of race and gender. Feminist theorists were essential for expanding the queer critique to gender, e.g. Eve Sedgwich, Judith Butler, Teresa de Lauretis. By disrupting the notion of fixed identities and breaking apart the dominant binaries of heterosexual/ homosexual, male/female, queer studies removed ideas of 'difference'. However, in doing so it negated differences that matter, in terms of power and privilege in the wider socio-political arena. Some of the identities and social connections that are negated are a source of support and survival against discrimination and oppression: 'in those stable categories and named communities whose histories have been structured by shared resistance to oppression, I find relative degrees of safety and security' (Cohen, 2005, 35). The voices of those from ethnic minorities are poorly represented (Cohen, 2005). Because of this queer theory is shaped by a white perspective: 'the assumptions made when constructing a theory, the determination of what is worth studying and what is not and the inferences drawn from empirical findings, will all be shaped by the culture of the theory makers' (Patel et al., 2000, 36).

Jay (2005, 107) paraphrases Johnson (2001) to suggest reasons why writers and theorists do not address whiteness:

1. 'Obliviousness/ignorance (they don't know what's going on).
2. Security/Complacency (they don't have to know what's going on).
3. Individualism (they think what's going on is a result of individual effort and/or merit, and that inequalities are therefore deserved).
4. Benefits (they don't want to lose what they gain because of what's going on).
5. Prejudice (they think they know what's going on and it offends them).
6. Fear (they are afraid that acknowledging what's going on will bring harm or loss to them)'.

By negating the issues of race, queer theorists do not reflect on the influence of their whiteness to their theorizing and hence how queer theory is a white Euro-American theory (Harper, 2005). This critique extends back to Foucault who discussed the formation of the homosexual identity with an unspoken assumption that his homosexuals were white, or else their racial identity was subsumed by their sexual identity so as to no longer be relevant (Ross, 2005). Goldman (1996), as a white bisexual woman, suggests that queer theorists shy away from discussing their whiteness because it positions them as the dominant majority. Carbado (2005) warns that dominant groups (in this case white queers) will 'discount the experiences of subordinate groups ... unless those experiences are authenticated or legitimized by a member of the dominant group' (p. 207). Similarly, Kilomba (2007) reminds us that 'academia is not a neutral location' ... but is largely a 'white space where Black people have been denied the privilege to speak'.

The activism side of queer politics (e.g. the work of Stonewall) also tends to be 'single issue' campaigns (e.g. adoption rights), with no discussion of the relevance or influence of these issues for black queers. Smith (1999) suggests that the lack of direct attention to racial oppression discourages black queers from joining these campaigns: 'I am particularly struck by the fact that for the most part queer theory and queer politics, which are currently so popular, offer neither substantial antiracist analysis nor practice' (Smith, 1999, 18).

A Black Queer Theory

A black queer theory finds its origins in the activism of the 1960s, 1970s and 1980s in the fight for equal rights for BMEs and women. Some of the strongest voices at this time were from feminists. From the late 1980s onwards, with the rise of the AIDS epidemic, a rich plethora of art and writing came from black queer men infected with the virus. More recently, there has been a refocus of desire and the black body.

Black Activism

The late 1960s saw the rise of the Civil Rights and Black Power movements in the US, and with it a push to develop 'black studies' in predominantly white higher education institutions. However, the heterosexual male leaders of these campaigns dictated the terms, which in uniting on race excluded all other identity categories, i.e. gender and sexuality (Johnson and Henderson, 2005). Fortunately, the 1970s and 1980s saw black feminists such as Audre Lorde, Angela Davies, Alice Walker, Cheryl Clarke, and Barbara Smith writing and campaigning until their voices broke through. Some of these women where also lesbians, who brought a challenge to heterosexism and homophobia within both the women's rights and civil rights movements (Johnson and Henderson, 2005).

> On the whole, Black British lesbians remained silent and isolated. We were required to break our identities into acceptable fragments: we were Black in Black groups, women in the women's movement and lesbians on the lesbian scene. There was no space to be whole, to be a Black lesbian. (Mason-John and Khambatta, 1993, 11)

This aspect of their writing was against the flow of the established heterosexist black discourse which positioned homosexuality as 'a "white disease" that had "infected" the black community' (Johnson and Henderson, 2005, 4). Denigration of queer identities within the black movement is oft based on the idea that to belong to a sexual minority group is a choice (which is controversial in itself), whereas one is black from birth: 'gays are pretenders to a throne of disadvantage that properly belongs to black[s]' (Gates, 1999, 25). Indeed, Mason-John and Khambatta (1993) suggest that the lack of acknowledgement of BME voices and experiences in queer theory is a denial of the existence of homosexuality within the black community: 'Because Black communities already experience discrimination on the grounds of race, colour and language, there is a fear among the heterosexual population that to admit the existence of a taboo like homosexuality would oppress them more, dragging them further into the gutter' (Mason-John and Khambatta, 1993, 21).

In contrast to this view, Lorde described the importance of the black movement as 'the very house of difference rather than the security of any one particular difference' (Lorde, 1982, 226). It is important to remember that there is no more homophobia in the black community than in heterosexist society in general: 'saying that homophobia is more prevalent in the Black community is like saying there are more Black men who rape' (Bellos, cited in Mason-John and Khambatta, 1993, 22).

Writing about black, colour and queer is more often than not authored by those individuals who identify in those terms, under those banners. The aim of writers such as Johnson (2005) is not only to fill a vacuum but to address a range of questions, among them: how can queer theory fulfil its promise of inclusively? The hope is that the exposition on the fundamental flaw exposed by the absence of BME voices could, in due course, help in queer theory's formation as a complete disciplinary 'subject'.

The Black Body and HIV/AIDS

HIV/AIDS disproportionately affects gay and bisexual men and transgender people from Black and minority ethnic communities, especially in the US with African American and Latino communities most affected (CDC, 2008). In the UK, Black and gay/bisexual men are the group most affected (HPA, 2006). Many services are set up to target one or other of these groups, without a recognition that they could be one of the same (an exception to this and an excellent example of service provision is written up by Zavuga, 2006). Dada (1990) highlights the racism that lies behind the uncritical acceptance by white gay writers that AIDS originated in Africa and that more black heterosexuals are infected. Dada suggests that this allows said writers to deflect 'blame' from the white gay community. In contrast to this lack of self-reflection, Black queer men in the US and UK have been writing, making art and being activists to addresses their personal experience of living with HIV (e.g. Gary Fisher; Gupta; Fani-Kayode).

The Black Body and Desire

The contradiction of the black body as a site for both desire and derision has been noted in sociological literature (Ford, 2008). An evaluation of the self, as viewed in the mirror, is never only a product of vision but of a perception that is coloured by the socio-political history of the self, in conjunction with racial and ethnic heritage, and the knowledge of others' perceptions of the self as a member of a specific racial/ethnic group. This kind of analytic viewing of the self is what Cooley (1902) referred to as 'the looking-glass self'.

The white colonial stereotype of a black man as an oversexed animal (and hence responsible for the spread of AIDS, as detailed above), and the transformation of his subjectship into an object – the penis – as material for fantasy (both heteroerotic and homoerotic) dates back to the times of slavery. Textual material suggestive of this bewitching allure is not only limited to the written text (novels), but is also embodied in the still images of Mapplethorpe (Mercer, 2002) and 'advertisements for Nike and other sport companies, the cinematic construction of Steven Spielberg's Armistad to the cover of black athlete's autobiographies, the black male torso as object of visual desire is everywhere' (Carrington, 2002, 21). Therefore, it is not surprising that black stereotypes are also held by black people. As Boykin (2002) posits, the black stereotype of a black man as 'uneducated and not as successful' (as a white man) is not uncommon. Racialized same-gendered desire can be considered a function of both racism (from non-black people) and internalized racism (within black people). Fetishization of the black body is another way in which racism is played out. Such fetishization also occurs for East Asian men, who are seen as feminine and subservient. Therefore, it is not only the East Asian man's body that is physically penetrated, but it is also metaphorically penetrated by the white gaze (Yancy, 2008). Thus, the white gaze may be able to *see* the black body because of its hypervisibility, but not *read* black subjectivity because of its invisibility (to the non-black person). However, if the black body does not conform to the fetish ideal, it needs to conform to the normative ideal, which is defined as white. Sandip Roy (1998) captures this view of the Asian body, even when viewed through the lens of another Asian (photographer): 'I had hoped that by controlling the camera we would be controlling the definition of erotic. But that definition had been set long ago by others; these pictures were just trying to live up to it' (p. 274).

The body is a significant cultural talisman in gay spaces. The commodity fetishization (cf. Marx, 1867/1988) of the body is a dominant theme in commercial gay venues/scenes (including cyberspace). Poon et al. (2005) found that in a sample of East and Southeast Asian men who used gay Internet chatrooms, many participants preferred white men. Whiteness here was used as a measure of attractiveness. The commodification of the body can be seen as a form of a (meat) market economy, whereby the low supply/availability of the white body to the Asian man creates a high demand for it. Thereby, other Asian men who have sex with men (MSM) are viewed as competitors for the limited number of white men (Poon et al., 2005). One recent British study (das Nair and Thomas, unpublished manuscript) found that over one-third of their sample of East and South Asian MSM felt that they were not desired because of their race or ethnicity. Of note here is that it was not only white men who they felt did not desire them, but also men from other BME groups and their own ethnic group.

The black body therefore is never a neutral space. It is gazed upon, perceived, acknowledged, touched, torched, desired and despised depending on the racial configurations of the self and the other, located in a given space and time. The politics that govern the use/abuse of the black body are closely intertwined with the constructions of race/ethnicity and sexuality. The textuality of such a weave is never complete or without fault, and can only be perceived like an Escher sketch, where background and foreground are both independent and interlocked, and constant switching between figure and ground is required to fully appreciate its complexity and scope.

Intersectionality: No Hierarchy of Oppression

Both Saint and Smith have commented on the existence of multiple identities and the assumption that one amongst them must take primacy:

> Afrocentrists in our community have chosen the term "black gay" to identify themselves. As they insist, black comes first. Interracialists in our community have chosen the term "gay black" to identify themselves. As they insist, gay comes first. Both groups' self-descriptions are ironically erroneous. It's not which word comes first that matters, but rather the grammatical context in which those words are used either as an adjective or as a noun. An adjective is a modifier of a noun. The former is dependent on the latter. (Saint, 1991, xix)

> Perhaps the most maddening question anyone can ask me is "Which do you put first: being black or being a woman, being black or being gay?" The underlying assumption is that I should prioritize one of my identities because one of them is actually more important than the rest or that I must arbitrarily choose one of them over the other for the sake of acceptance in one particular community. (Smith, 1999, 15)

The imposition of a hierarchy of oppression has lead many queers to negotiate and manipulate identity labels. Labels have the power to potentially dilute self-identity when multiple identities, such as woman, black, lesbian and mother, are denied visibility through a singular dominantly assigned label. Labels can persuade and validate, or condemn and exclude. They can invoke fear and pride, offer acceptance or denial. Adopting a new label can be transformative, changing not only self-perception but also how others may shift their perceptions and views. Because of this queers have not casually accepted the labels that are assigned to them (Eyben and Moncrieff, 2007).

Any project that attempts to explore the intersections between identities is therefore essentialist, and requires the grouping and categorizing of people based on various dimensions. While some identities are self-ascribed, others are imposed upon individuals by society. For instance, a woman may consider herself 'heterosexual', but may be labelled as being a 'butch lesbian' purely on the basis of her demeanour and appearance, which society may deem as falling outside the norms of femininity. However, the problem with such categorizations is that they can never be complete or static, and their relative nature makes them volatile. Any queering project, therefore, becomes another subjugating force if it compels people to conform to the narrow confines of *an* identity, or requires them to rank-order their multiple identities, without exploring the process or contexts in which such an ordering takes place.

There are intersections of identities that have a summative effect of disadvantaging individuals who find themselves in multiple positions that society has deemed subordinate: 'As a black, lesbian, feminist, socialist, poet, mother of two including one boy and a member of an interracial couple, I usually find myself part of some group in which the majority defines me as deviant, difficult, inferior or just plan "wrong"' (Lorde, 1999, 306). However, there are times where these intersections can be advantageous. Rather than considering the additive/summative nature of disenfranchisement caused by belonging to multiple categories of minorityhood, much more can be gleaned by examining the faultlines at which these minority identities are performed and contested. Fisher (2003) refers to her experiences of being a lesbian, belonging to an ethnic minority, and the manner in which multiple minority identities actually permits one to negotiate sexuality in ways which would not traditionally be considered as appropriate or proud. She suggests cultural hybridity encourages people to use the 'closet' in creative ways to achieve this. She draws on Michel de Certeau's (1984) idea of tactics that queer immigrants apply to their daily micro-practices. She argues that 'contrary to a popularized valorization of queer "outness", there is a great deal of power in the oscillation between visibility and invisibility' (p. 171). There is a pertinent point being made here: the models of coming out, affirmative gay life, and gay 'pride' may not always be applicable to black queer people (cf. Exercise 8.3 previously). In Fisher's (2003) case, she elucidates this creativity when describing a birthday party where people from various (queer and not queer) communities were attending. During such social situations she speaks of the deployment of 'a number of performative micro-operations ... including silences, fibs, contrived personal details, exaggerated gestures, seemingly innocent facial expressions, cautious glances, polite nods of the head, and carefully orchestrated seating positions 'to live life in the hyphen' (p. 177).

These imaginative cultural performances may at times be at variance with prescribed ways of being queer. This is because most models of coming out have not factored in the race/ethnicity element and therefore do not take into account how black queer people can navigate with and through their multiple identities. Following from this, these models therefore cannot be applied directly to non-white queer individuals (who may or may not identify as lesbian or gay). In fact, there are potential threats and dangers associated with coming out in certain contexts (Cole Wilson and Allen, 1994). Thus, when examining the differences between various metaminorities (minorities within a minority population, das Nair, 2006), we need to move on from asking what configuration of minority statuses are more 'worse off' than others (Purdie-Vaughns and Eibach, 2008), to exploring how subjugation because of these statuses are derived, inculcated, propagated, and maintained and how these individuals creatively use these multiple identities to celebrate these differences holistically.

Many people from ethnic minority groups who love and/or have sex with someone of the same gender would not use the label lesbian or gay; this might be because the terms are associated with the West or with danger. For example, the term 'lesbian' can be associated with feminism and used to make a political statement rather than just to express a sexual/emotional preference (Reinfelder, 1996). The term 'lesbian' has also been seen as a white term, with alternative words available in different languages and cultures, such as Zami, dyke, wicker, khush (Reinfelder, 1996). In addition, the term bisexuality may not be used by people who live a primarily heterosexual life, while also loving and being sexual with people of the same gender. Reinfelder (1996) suggests that the absence of a label might actually make same-sex love and sexuality more tolerable in some communities (e.g. for women who are married and have children but also have women lovers. Sex is equated with the penis and so 'no harm is seen in two women sleeping together' (p. 3)).

If we recognize the multiple and intersecting parts of people's identities, there can be no hierarchy of oppression. Such a politic is possible and captured within the black feminist group, the Combahee River Collective's opening position statement: 'we are actively committed to struggling against racial, sexual, heterosexual, and class oppression and see as our particular task the development of integrated analysis and practice based upon the fact that the major systems of oppression are interlocking. This synthesis of these oppressions creates the conditions of our lives' (Smith, 1983, 272).

The rejection of categorical labels to describe sexuality fits within queer theory, which replaces 'socially named and presumably stable categories of sexual expression with a new fluid movement among and between forms of sexual behavior' (Cohen, 2005, 22–23). Thus by resisting a fixed definition, the ability to be categorized and deemed 'other' or deviant from the accepted norm is resisted (Cohen, 2005), and the power and privilege inherent in such categorization is highlighted. However, as previously discussed, 'queer' runs the risk of becoming the new monolithic identifier negating other aspects of selfhood. In addition, the rejection of labels which contain power, such as 'white', negates reflection on the positions and privileges they allow. In negotiating and flexing the labels available and interactions between them, a critical analysis of the power present or absent within remains important.

Conclusion

There is no a single fixed black, white or queer identity; these are social constructs that shift over time and place, in line with in and out groups and the allocation of power and resources. We have argued that for those denied access to this power, privilege and resources there is no hierarchy of oppression. We join the voices of previous writers (e.g. Smith, Lorde, Johnson) in suggesting that to make single-identity issues a focus of resistance is to ill-serve ourselves and others with dangerous consequences. This move away from a focus on a single identity marker fits neatly within the thesis of queer theory. However, we warn that this does not mean that multiple identity markers are not always present, those in the foreground depending on the current context, and their interaction should remain examined. There is heterogeneity of experiences that black and white queer people have on the basis of their sexuality and/or race. The intersections of multiple minority identities could both be a site of (further) subjugation/domination or an opportunity to negotiate creative ways of being both black/white and queer. We suggest that further analysis of race and its interaction with queer theory is necessary to deconstruct the mainly unexamined frame of whiteness and incorporate the voices of blackness.

Further Reading

Davy, K. (1997), 'Outing whiteness: A feminist lesbian project', in M. Hill (ed.), *Whiteness: A Critical Reader* (New York: New York University Press).

Dyer, R. (1997), *White* (London: Routledge).

Ignatiev, N. (1996), *How the Irish Became White* (London: Routledge).

Johnson, E. and M. Henderson (eds) (2005), *Black Queer Studies: A Critical Anthology* (NC: Duke University Press).

Morrison, T. (1992), *Playing in the Dark: Whiteness and the Literary Imagination* (Cambridge, MA: Harvard University Press).

Schuhmann, A. and M. Wright (eds) (2008), *Blackness and Sexualities* (Münster: Lit Verlag).

Yancy, G. (2008), *Black Bodies, White Gazes: The Continuing Significance of Race* (New York: Rowman and Littlefield).

References

Bartlett, A., Smith, G. and King, M. (2009), 'The response of mental health professionals to clients seeking help to change or redirect same-sex sexual orientation', *BMC Psychiatry*, 9, 11.

Bergman, D. (1991), *Gaiety Transfigured: Gay Self-Representation in American Literature* (Madison: University of Wisconsin Press).

Bhui, K., Stansfeld, S., Hull, S., Priebe, S., Mole, F. and Feder, G. (2003), 'Ethnic variations in pathways to and use of specialist mental health services in the UK: Systematic review', *British Journal of Psychiatry*, 182, 105–116.

Boykin, K. (2002), *No Blacks Allowed*. Retrieved 18.04.2009 from Temenos <www.temenos.net/articles/12-23-04.shtml>.

Bright, D. (ed.) (1998), *The Passionate Camera: Photography and Bodies of Desire* (London and New York: Routledge).

Brod, H. (1989), 'Work clothes and leisure suits: The class basis and bias of the men's movement', in M.S. Kimmel and M. Messner (eds), *Men's Lives* (New York: Macmillan).

Carbado, D.W. (2005), 'Privilege', in E.P. Johnson and M.G. Henderson (eds), *Black Queer Studies: A Critical Anthology* (Durham, DC: Duke University Press).

Carrington, B. (2002), *'Race', Representation and the Sporting Body* (Brighton: University of Brighton).

Centre for Disease Control and Prevention (CDC) (2008), *HIV/AIDS Among African Americans* (Atlanta: Department of Health and Human Sciences).

Certeau, M. de (1984), *The Practice of Everyday Life*. Translated by Steven Rendall (Berkeley, CA: University of California Press).

Cohen, C.J. (2005), 'Punks, bulldaggers, and welfare queens: The radical potential of queer politics', in E.P. Johnson and M.G. Henderson (eds), *Black Queer Studies: A Critical Anthology* (Durham, DC: Duke University Press).

Cohen, C.J. and Jones, T. (1999), 'Fighting homophobia versus challenging heterosexism: "The Failure to Transform" revisited', in E. Brandt (ed.), *Dangerous Liaisons: Blacks, Gays and the Struggle for Equality* (New York: Norton and Company).

Cole Wilson, O. and Allen, C. (1994), 'The black perspective', in E. Healey and A. Mason (eds), *Stonewall 25: The Making of the Lesbian and Gay Community in Britain* (London: Virago Press).

Cooley, C.H. (1902), *Human Nature and the Social Order* (New York: Scribner's).

Dada, M. (1990), 'Race and the AIDS agenda', in T. Boffin and S. Gupta (eds), *Ecstatic Antibodies: Resisting the AIDS Mythology* (London: Rivers Oram Press).

das Nair, R. (2006), *Metaminorities and Mental Health: Pathways of Vulnerability for Black and Minority Ethnic Queer Folk*, Inter-Disciplinary Net: Oxford <http://www.inter-disciplinary.net/ci/sexuality/s2/nair%20paper.pdf>.

das Nair, R. and Thomas, S. (n.d.), 'Politics of Desire: Exploring the Ethnicity/Sexuality Intersectionality in South Asian and East Asian Men Who Have Sex With Men' (MSM). Unpublished manuscript.

Derrida, J. (1978), 'Cogito and the History of Madness', from *Writing and Difference*. Translated by A. Bass. (London and New York: Routledge).

Eyben, R. and Moncrieff, J. (eds) (2007), *The Power of Labelling: How and Why People's Categories Matter* (London: Earthscan).

Fisher, D. (2003), 'Immigrant closets: Tactical-micro-practices-in-the-hyphen', *Journal of Homosexuality*, 45(2/3/4), 171–192.

Floyd-James, D. (2001), *Who is Black? One Nation's Definition* (Pennsylvania: University Press).

Ford, K. (2008), 'Gazing into a distorted looking glass: Masculinity, femininity, appearance ideals, and the black body', *Sociology Compass*, 2/3, 1096–1114.

Ford, R.T. (2007), 'What's queer about race?', *South Atlantic Quarterly*, 106(3), 477–484.

Gates, H.L. (1999), 'Blacklash?', in E. Brandt (ed.), *Dangerous Liaisons: Blacks, Gays and the Struggle for Equality* (New York: Norton and Company).

Goldman, R. (1996), 'Who is queer?', in B. Beemyn and M. Eliason (eds), *Queer Studies: A Lesbian, Gay, Bisexual and Transgender Anthology* (New York: New York University Press).

Gupta, S. (2003), *A World Without Pity* [Short documentary film].

Harper, P.D. (2005), 'The evidence of felt intuition: Minority experience, everyday life, and critical speculative knowledge', in E.P. Johnson and M.G. Henderson (eds), *Black Queer Studies: A Critical Anthology* (Durham, DC: Duke University Press).

Haymes, S. (1996), 'Race, repression, and the politics of crime and punishment in the bell curve', in J. Kincheloe, S. Steinberg and A. Gresson (eds), *Measured Lies: The Bell Curve Examined* (New York: St Martin's Press).

HPA (2006), *HIV, AIDS and Sexually Transmitted Infections in the UK* (London: Health Protection Agency).

Jay, G. (1997), 'Taking multiculturalism personally: Ethnos and ethos in the classroom', in G. Jay, *American Literature and the Culture Wars* (Ithaca, NY: Cornell University Press).

Jay, G. (2005), 'Whiteness studies and the multicultural literature classroom', *MELUS*, 30(2), 99–121.

Johnson, A.G. (2001), *Privilege, Power and Difference* (New York: McGraw-Hill).

Johnson, E.P. (2005), '"Quare" studies, or (almost) everything I know about queer studies I learned from my grandmother', in E.P. Johnson and M.G. Henderson (eds), *Black Queer Studies: A Critical Anthology* (Durham, DC: Duke University Press).

Johnson, E.P. and Henderson, M.G. (2005), 'Introduction: Queering black studies "Quaring" queer studies', in E.P. Johnson and M.G. Henderson (eds), *Black Queer Studies: A Critical Anthology* (Durham, DC: Duke University Press).

Keating, F., Robertson, D., McCulloch, A. and Francis, E. (2000), *Breaking the Circles of Fear: A Review of the Relationship between Mental Health Services and the African and Caribbean Communities* (London: The Sainsbury Centre for Mental Health).

Kilomba, G. (2007), 'Africans in academia: Diversity in adversity' <http://www.africafiles.org/article.asp?ID=15961>.

Kincheloe, J.L. (1999), 'The struggle to define and reinvent whiteness: A pedagogical analysis', *College Literature* 26(3), 162–195.

Kutchins, H. and Kirk, S.A. (1999), *Making us Crazy* (London: Constable).

Lorde, A. (1982), *Zami: A New Spelling of My Name* (Watertown, MA: Persephone Press).

Lorde, A. (1999), 'There is no hierarchy of oppressions', in E. Brandt (ed.), *Dangerous Liaisons: Blacks, Gays and the Struggle for Equality* (New York: Norton and Company).

Lloyd, P. and Moodley, P. (1992), 'Psychotropic medication and ethnicity: An inpatient survey', *Social Psychiatry and Psychiatric Epidemiology* 27(2), 95–101.

Lucal, B. (1996), 'Oppression and privilege: Toward a relational conceptualisation of race', *Teaching Sociology* 24(3), 245–255.

McIntosh, P. (1997), 'White Privilege: Unpacking the invisible knapsack', in B. Schneider (ed.), *Race* (New York: Three Rivers Press).

Mason-John, V. and Khambatta, A. (1993), *Lesbians Talk: Making Black Waves*. London: Scarlet Press.

Marx, K. (1867/1988), *Capital*, Vol. I (London: Penguin).

Mercer, K. (2002), 'Skin head sex thing: Racial difference and the homoerotic imaginary', in R. Adams and D. Sagran (eds), *The Masculinity Studies Reader* (Oxford: Wiley-Blackwell).

Moya, P. (1997), 'Postmodernism, "realism" and the politics of identity: Cherrie Moraga and Chicano Feminism', in M.J. Alexander and C.T. Mohanty (eds), *Feminist Genealogies, Colonial Legacies, Democratic Futures* (New York: Routledge).

Ng, V. (1997), 'Race matters', in A. Medhurst and S.R. Munt (eds), *Lesbian and Gay Studies: A Critical Introduction* (London: Cassell).

Patel, N., Bennett, E., Dennis, M., Dosanjh, N., Mantani, A., Miller, A. and Nadirshaw, Z. (2000), *Clinical Psychology, 'Race' and Culture: A Training Manual* (Leicester: BPS).

Poon, K.-L., Ho, P.T.-T., Wong, J.P.-H., Wong, G. and Lee, R. (2005), 'Psychosocial experiences of East and Southeast Asian men who use gay internet chatrooms in Toronto: An implication for HIV/AIDS prevention', *Ethnicity and Health* 10(2), 145–167.

Purdie-Vaughns, V. and Eibach, R.P. (2008), 'Intersectional invisibility: The distinctive advantages and disadvantages of multiple subordinate-group identities', *Sex Roles* 59, 377–391.

Reinfelder, M. (1996), *Amazon to Zami* (London: Cassell).

Roediger, D.R. (2005), *Working Towards Whiteness: How American's Immigrants became White. The Strange Journey from Ellis Island to the Suburbs* (New York: Basic Books).

Ross, M.R. (2005), 'Beyond the closet as raceless paradigm', in E.P. Johnson and M.G. Henderson (eds), *Black Queer Studies: A Critical Anthology* (Durham, DC: Duke University Press).

Roy, S. (1998), 'Mapping My Desire: Hunting Down the Male Erotic in India and America', in D. Atkins (ed.), *Looking Queer: Body Image and Identity in Lesbian, Bisexual, Gay, and Transgender Communities* (New York: Haworth Press).

Saint, A. (ed.) (1991), *The Road Before Us: 100 Gay Black Poets* (New York: Galiens).

Smith, B. (ed.) (1983), *Home Girls: A Black Feminist Anthology* (New York: Women of Color Press).

Smith, D. (1999), 'Black and gays: Healing the great divide', in E. Brandt (ed.), *Dangerous Liaisons: Blacks, Gays and the Struggle for Equality* (New York: Norton and Company).

Yancy, G. (2008), *Black Bodies, White Gazes: The Continuing Significance of Race* (Lanham, MD: Rowman and Littlefield Publishers).

Zavuga, J. (2006), 'HIV prevention work with African men who have sex with men: Interventions at the community level', *Lesbian and Gay Psychology Review* 7(3), 282–286.

Zetzer, H.A. (2005), 'White out: Privilege and its problems', in S.K. Anderson and V.A. Middleton (eds), *Explorations in Privilege, Oppression and Diversity* (Belmont, CA: Thomson Brooks/Cole).

Chapter 7

'I Did It My Way …':
Relationship Issues for Bisexual People

Christian Klesse

Introduction

Recent developments in sexual politics have brought concerns around non-heterosexual relationships onto the public agenda. Since the 1980s increasing energy has been dedicated by activists to campaigning around relational rights for same-sex partners (Weeks et al. 2001). The struggles were propelled by the injustices at the heart of heteronormative state practices and hegemonic cultural values, which only grant recognition and rights to relationships which follow the scripts provided by white middle class heterosexual coupledom. The demand for same-sex marriage rights (or civil partnership rights) has occupied the public debate on cultural values and jurisdiction in many countries (Heaphy 2007, Wintemute and Andenæs 2000). Even if the issue of same-sex marriage rights still is subject to heated controversy, it is evident that the introduction of civil partnership schemes in many legal systems has brought some forms of non-heterosexual bonding closer into the realm of citizenship proper (Bell and Binnie 2000, Richardson 2000). Gay and lesbian partnerships are visible to a much stronger degree across the media and various genres within popular culture (Gamson 1998, Cossman 2007).

Yet the growing recognition for some forms of non-heterosexual intimacy is limited to certain kinds of attachment, which draw their ultimate legitimation from the universalised value of the monogamous long term bond based on romantic sentiment (Berlant and Warner 1998, Klesse 2007a). The preoccupation with lesbian and gay couples and families has not been confined to the political and legal spheres. Counselling and self-help resources have been provided to address the problems and concerns of same-sex couples. Yet this material, too, usually only addresses a limited range of relationship issues due to its primary concern with a narrow model of coupledom (Klesse 2007b). There is a widespread assumption that partners in a same-sex relationship do also identify as gay or lesbian. Yet sexual behaviour and identification does not necessarily match ready-made categorisations of sexual orientation. While the relationship concerns of white middle class gay men and lesbians have gained somewhat more attention over recent years, the awareness of other forms of desire, identification and affectionate bonds is still quite limited. Bisexuality is a case in point. There is a striking absence of research into bisexual relationships and intimacies. The lack of awareness around and education on bisexuality among counsellors and psychotherapists has serious implications for the service provision for bisexuals and their partners (Neal and Davis 2000b).[1] Some of the problems many bisexuals face in their intimate lives may be very similar to the ones encountered by people of other sexual identification. Yet others are quite specific to bisexual lives. In this chapter, I explore some of the issues which are more closely tied into cultural practices and understandings around bisexuality. I focus on issues around identification, bi-negativity (or biphobia), kin work, lack of support networks, gender relations and sexual practices. I develop themes identified by previous research and draw on my own study into bisexual intimacies, which I conducted as part of a larger project into contemporary discourses on non-monogamy (Klesse 2007a).

What is Bisexuality? Who is a Bisexual?

Bisexuality is very difficult to define. Both within the academic literature and popular culture different understandings of bisexuality intermingle. Bisexuality is a Western concept on sexuality, which emerged in a close interrelationship with the sexual categories homosexuality and heterosexuality in nineteenth century attempts to classify human sexual types and conditions (Weeks 1990, Bristow 1997). While it is generally assumed that people are either heterosexual or homosexual, bisexuality has played a more ambiguous role. Although it has been an active element in most theories on sexuality, it has rarely been seen as an authentic sexuality in its own right (Hemmings 2002, Angelides 2000). Bisexuality has assumed different meanings since its first inception, when it was supposed to stand in for an intermediate state of sexual differentiation in the development of biological organisms (Storr 1999). Today the most common meaning of the term bisexuality is a form of desire, in which erotic attraction is not limited to one gender. This understanding is expressed in at least two competing narratives. In the first one, bisexuality stands for a desire for both men and women. In this account, bisexuality is framed as an inherently dual orientation. In the second

---

1   It has taken a long time until the validation of bisexual identities has been considered an integral part of critical debates on heteronormativity and heterosexism in counselling and therapy (Davies and Neal 2000, 2003, Neal and Davis 2000a, Moon 2008). Yet detailed knowledge is scarce and a specific bisexual perspective is hardly to be found. When Dominic Davies and Charles Neal edited the first volume of their trilogy on 'gay affirmative' therapy in 1996 they did acknowledge bisexual identities and the prevalence of biphobia. Yet in the absence of research into bisexual psychology they decided to subsume bisexuality within a lesbian and gay framework (Davies and Neal 2003, Davies 2003). This tendency is also revealed in the act of labelling their approach of a person-centred therapeutic practice with gay men, lesbians, bisexuals and transgender people as a 'gay affirmative' approach (Davies and Neal 2000b – Perspectives – Intro). Only one of the volumes published in the year 2000 contains a more complex discussion of bisexuality and counselling (Oxley and Lucius 2000).

narrative, bisexuality is presented as a form of desire which does not discriminate in terms of gender. Here sexual desire is not determined by a gendered preference for object choice (which does not mean that it is entirely free of gendered meanings) (Hemmings 2002, Rodriguez Rust 2000a-binary). This interpretation of bisexuality avoids the trap of framing sexual desire in terms of a dichotomy (even if, arguably, the term bi-sexuality linguistically reproduces this binary). It is often based on a proactive recognition that the concepts of maleness and femaleness (or masculinity and femininity) do not exhaust the full range of gender identities. It does therefore not paradigmatically exclude transgender realities (cf. Califia 1997, Nestle et al. 2002, Whittle 2002). The common definition of bisexuality as desire for men and women or a kind of pan-sexuality is often still over-layered by other meanings derived from history. It is not uncommon to find in 20th texts century on bisexuality references to androgyny or gender identity ambiguity, which stem from previous definitions of bisexuality as psychic (if not physical) hermaphroditism (Angelides 2000).

While it is difficult to define bisexuality, it is even a trickier task to decide when we can talk of a person as being bisexual. Even if we stay with the most common definition described above, different criteria may be considered in approaching this question. Is it a person's desire which renders them bisexual, as for example their capacity to desire men and women (or 'people' – irrespective of the sexed state of their bodies)? Or is a person only bisexual, if he or she maintains concurrent relationships with both men and women? If we assume this to be the case, does this person then stop to be bisexual once he or she loses their involvement with representatives of one or even both genders? (cf. Zinik 1985). Or is a person only bisexual, if they identify as bisexual. Personally, I hold the view that self-identity should be the ultimate criterion on this question, in particular in person affirmative approaches to counselling and therapy (Davies 2003, Neal and Davies 2000b).

Many self-identified bisexuals hold the view that their identity is *not* dependent on their current relationship status or their sexual practice in any particular period of their life. Yet, unfortunately, many find their identities interrogated, if they do not maintain visible relationships to men and women at a particular period of their lives. This is a result of the pervasive belief that authentic bisexuality is impossible – apart from (situational) expression in multi-gendered multiple partnership constellations (Klesse 2007a). These problems of definition often directly result from the ambiguous and contingent role which bisexuality plays in wider discourses on human sexuality. In this chapter I am primarily concerned with people who identify as bisexual or reference bisexuality in their identification. There is great diversity within and around 'bisexual' identity narratives, as evidenced frequent usage of 'hyphenated' identity labels, such as for example 'bi-dyke', 'queer-identified bisexual', 'bi-curious heterosexual', etc. (cf. Ault 1999, Bower et al. 2002). Sexual identity labels may further intersect with political, ethnic and class identities (Jordan 1996, Ellis 1999). I suppose, even people who do not identify with the label bisexuality at all (for whatever reason) but who are open about their sexual attraction to people of different genders may find elements of the discussion in this chapter relevant. Society tends to find bisexuality challenging – whether it presents itself as a form of identification or non-closeted forms of behaviour.

'Relationship Issues' and Sexual Identification

There is a certain risk associated with writing an article about 'relationship problems' for bisexual people. This is because non-heterosexual relationships have been represented as deviant, pathological, problem-ridden and doomed to fail throughout decades of scientific writing (Weeks et al. 1996, Carrington 1999). Queer or queer-friendly scholars therefore dedicated efforts to challenging the common misrepresentation of non-heterosexual relationship lives as unsettled, fragile, clichéd and bizarre. This is why we find so many comparative studies, which show that there is no difference in relationship satisfaction between gay and lesbian and heterosexual relationships (cf. Kurdek 1995, Peplau et al. 1997, Weeks et al. 1996). As I said earlier, bisexuals have usually been absent from these research scenarios. According to Paula Rodriguez Rust (2000b), only one 'genre' of research looked at bisexuals and their intimate partnerships before the HIV/AIDS epidemic triggered a newish interest into bisexuality from an entirely epidemiological point of view. In the 1980s a small range of studies appeared which looked at so-called 'mixed-orientation marriages'. These studies focused on the question how married heterosexual partners manage to cope with their realisation that their spouse starts to assume a gay, lesbian (or bisexual) identity. The big topics of this research perspective were crisis management, adaptation and/or separation (cf. Rodriguez Rust 2000b, Klesse 2007a). Of course, it is not in my interest to reinforce the misguided representation that bisexual relationships (or any other forms of non-heterosexual intimacies) are inherently problematic or problem-ridden. Even if still limited in numbers, contemporary research attests to a diverse, innovative and satisfying relationship culture crated by bisexuals and their intimate and sexual partners (Rust 1996a, Weinberg et al. 1994, George 1993, Atkins 2002, Klesse 2007a).

Moreover, all people – irrespective of their sexual identities – face challenges and problems in their relationships. To give just a few examples: Economic hardship and scarcity of resources affects relationships and families across differences in terms of sexuality. Differences in income and social and cultural capital create divisions in lesbian, gay, bisexual and queer families as much as in heterosexual relationships (Carrington 1999, Hennessy 1995).[2] Partners and families of various sexualities may face compulsory separation due to restrictive legislation around citizenship

------

2   The absence of a systematic address of class issues in the literature on same-sex relationships reveals the extent to which debates about relational rights reflect an agenda which speaks most to the concern of white middle class people (Lehr 1999, Cohen 2001, Stychin 2003).

and immigration status.[3] Many problems within relationships extend to bonds of all kinds of sexualities, too. It has been widely documented that abuse is a problem not only in straight relationships, but extends to queer intimacies of all kinds (Leventhal and Lundy 1999, Island and Lettelier 1992). Relationships may be unsettled by psychological problems of individual partners or family members. Separation difficulties and custody conflicts occur across the whole range of family diversity – even if frequently dealt with in distinct ways by individual judges (Monk 2009). An unequal division of labour between partners, whether on the level of emotionality or in the larger context of reproductive work may cause problems in relationships. Although research indicates that role expectations in this area are clearly gendered (Jamieson 1998), it has been established that lesbian, gay and bisexual relationships are not usually egalitarian either (Carrington 1999). This list could be expanded. I name these examples to demonstrate that in many regards relationship issues for bisexual people do overlap with the ones for people of other sexual preferences and identities. Yet at the same time, there are also issues which are more specific to bisexual lives. In the following, I will concentrate on potential problems related to bisexual identification and the various effects of biphobic representation and practice – both within wider society and the gay and lesbian 'communities'.

Bisexuality and Identification

Research indicates that many people collect sexual experiences with men and women across their life course. A much smaller number of people actively identify as bisexual (Fox 1996, Paul 1997). There are manifold explanations for this. The persisting stigma of bisexuality as a non-heterosexual identity is a highly relevant one (Ochs 1996). Research into bisexual identities suggests that identification processes around bisexuality are often complex and uneven. Bi-identified people present coming-out narratives, which contain more references to identity-changes than self-stories of other-identified individuals (Rust 1996b). Bisexuals often assume a bisexual identity or come out as 'bisexuals' comparatively late in their biography (Fox 1996). Far from seeing these specifities of identification around

---

3   In the absence of civil partnership legislation queer relationships were denied access to an important route towards legalising residence of a non-EU partner, if they wished to live together in the UK. Same-sex relationships have been clearly discriminated against in family reunion schemes in many countries (Binnie 1997, Simmons 2007). The introduction of civil partnership legislation in many EU countries has altered this situation to a certain extent. Yet problems even persist for partnered EU citizens due to the uneven legalisation of same-sex partnerships across the EU (Ytterberg 2008). Inequalities and injustices further result from the absence of an effective implementation of transgender rights in EU countries (Whittle 2002). At the same time it could be argued that the primary mechanisms of exclusion operates along the lines of a racialised politics of granting citizenship (Kofman et al. 2000, Solomos 2003).

bisexuality as deficiency or an inherent indecisiveness, many researchers argue that the non-linearity of bisexual identity narratives reflects the construction of bisexuality as a transient, immature and ultimately non-liveable identity in wider social discourses on sexuality (Rust 1996b, Fox 1996).

If we assume a social constructionist perspective and understand identity as a temporary mooring or the posting of landmarks in a changing sexual landscape, the language available for identification and the conditions for articulating a particular identity become of paramount importance (Rust 1996b). Poststructuralist theories on identification have furthered some of the above mentioned insights of social constructionist models (Hemmings 2002, Bi Academic Intervention 1997). Poststructuralist theory emphasises the fragility and conditionality and historicity of any act of identification (Hall 1992, 1996) and thus helps to de-pathologise identity-changes. An understanding of identification in the light of poststructuralist assumptions directs our attention even more to the cultural processes around any particular social or sexual identity. If to identify means to claim an identity position shaped by discourses (Laclau 1990, Howarth 2000, Howarth and Stavrakakis 2000), it is no surprise at all that the ambiguity of discourses around bisexuality have far-reaching effects on individual identification processes. Even if an identity position of 'bisexual' is intelligible and available, it is continuously undermined in anti-bisexual common sense perceptions which reduce this position to a 'phase', an erratic delusion or self-denial (of a truly gay or lesbian identity).

Of course, other non-heterosexual identities, too, meet the habitual onslaughts of heteronormative forces of erasure (Butler 1990, 1993, Sedgwick 1993). Yet claiming a bisexual identity means claiming an identity which is generally cast as being no proper identity at all (Bell 1994). The scarcity of visible or supportive (bisexual) culture adds to this problematic. Although bisexual politics resulted in an increased awareness around bisexual issues, there are still relatively few bisexual networks or organisations and bisexual spaces are mostly temporary and transient. Bi-identified people primarily socialise in lesbian and gay or queer space, in which they frequently remain invisible (Hemmings 2002). It is against the backdrop of these factors that many bisexuals who are in a monogamous long term relationship (with a person of their own or a distinct gender) find it difficult to maintain a distinctive bisexual identity. Gay and lesbian identities gain stabilisation through a cultural politics of visibility, something which is not possible (or available) to the same extent in many bisexual relationship contexts. Assumptions on the transitory nature of bisexual identity among friends (and maybe even among partners) creates a further set of problems. If a bisexual person, who has lived in a largely lesbian, gay or bisexual context, enters a relationship with an other-sex partner, this may be perceived as a cop-out and a retreat into a sphere of heterosexual privilege by many people in that network (Valverde 1985, Oxley and Lucius 2000). In lesbian feminist circles such reactions are often particularly pronounced due to the strong politicisation of gendered partner choice in political lesbianism (cf. Rust 1995, Ault 1996, Stein 1997).

If a person who identifies as bisexual enters a same-sex relationship, many may be relieved and settle in the belief that this person has finally come to terms with his/her (truly) lesbian or gay desire. In both scenarios, bisexual identification is undermined and can only be maintained (if that is the person's wish) through assertion. Yet insisting on a bisexual identity in a monogamous relationship with either a gay male or a lesbian-identified person may cause a variety of other problems. Since identifying as bisexual emphasises the capacity to desire men and women and embraces this capacity as a feature of character which this person does not want to discard or deny, the myth of monogamy as a unique life-long bond between two partners who have been made for each other is difficult to maintain (Rust 1996b, Ault 8). Monogamous (non-bisexual) partners often create anxieties, if a bisexual person insists on maintaining a (public) bisexual identity. The fact that bisexuals are often perceived to be inherently non-monogamous or promiscuous adds to this problem. The over-sexualisation of bisexuals in the common imagination is a central feature of biphobic representations (Udis-Kessler 1996). Of course, many bi-identified people are in relationships with bi-identified partners, a situation which renders some of these problems less likely to emerge (cf. Weinberg et al. 1994, Queen 1996). Moreover, some bisexual people may wish to live in relationships which are based on a principle of non-monogamy, an issue which will explore in more detail later in this chapter. My main interest in this section was to illustrate that claiming a bisexual identity may cause insecurities, anxieties and problems in certain relationship contexts. These problems are largely the result of the construction of bisexuality as an inherently problematic if not impossible identity and sexuality. The denial and devaluation of bisexuality is commonly referred to as biphobia. In the following section, I will expand on my discussion how biphobia may complicate intimate and sexual relationships of bi-identified people.

Dealing with Biphobia: Stigma, Erasure and Bisexual Intimacies

Non-heterosexual identities and sexualities have been systematically devalued, misrepresented and oppressed in most societies for many centuries. Legal decriminalisation has been uneven and frequently does not provide a halt to the reproduction of stereotypes and social discrimination (cf. Evans 1993, Stychin 2003). This is why the price for coming out with a stigmatised non-heterosexual identity can still be high, depending on the social positioning and cultural networks of a person (Mercer and Isaac 1988). The denigration of gay male, lesbian, bisexual and other queer identities works through various distinct repertoires of representations, which are further mediated by dominant ideas on race, ethnicity and class (Haritaworn et al. 2006). People who analysed the oppression and marginalisation of bisexuality have argued that the expression of bisexual behaviours and identities tends to be regulated through a set of discourses and practices which only overlap to a certain extent with the ones directed against gay men and lesbians. Biphobia, they argue, is different from homophobia or lesbophobia (Ochs 1996, Paul 1997, cf. Adam 1998). Biphobia (or bi-negativity) stands for the various forms of exclusion and oppression experienced by bisexuals in diverse areas of their existence. It consists in prejudiced behaviour, stereotypical representation, practices of discrimination, erasure (denial, authoritative incorporation or assimilation) and acts of violence stimulated by the above mentioned attitudes and believes. Biphobia is pervasive in the sense that it is not limited to certain identity positions or cultural terrains. Heterosexuals, gay men, lesbians and – yes – bisexuals, too, may hold negative and views on bisexuals and bisexuality. Every form of power leaves its traces in the minds and psyche of the people who are denigrated through it. Very much alike to the adaptation of the term 'internalised homophobia' by the lesbian and gay movement (Hodges and Hutter 1974), bisexual activists and theorists have explored the effects of bi-negativity on the self-image and self-representation of bisexual people.

Amanda Udis Kessler (1996) has provided a comprehensive discussion of common anti-bi stereotypes. The common assumption that 'there's no such thing as bisexual identity' is a prime example of 'bisexual erasure'. It further mobilises a range of negative images which depict bisexuals as confused, indecisive, deluded or cowards. Bisexual are seen as 'fence-sitters', i.e. people who cannot make up their mind to join one of the proper parties or to face their true essential self. Other stereotypes elaborate sexual themes. Bisexuals tend to be represented as are excessive, promiscuous and incapable of monogamy. There is the common assumption that bisexuals do have be in con-current relationships with each gender in order to be happy of satisfied. Anti-bisexual promiscuity discourses have plugged into HIV/AIDS anxieties and given rise to a quite specific set of discourse, which describe bisexual men and women as the bridges of transmission between high-risk groups and the 'heterosexual community'. Thus, bisexuals have been stigmatised as 'AIDS carriers' (Weinberg et al. 1994, Klesse 2007a, Gorna 1996). Bisexuals have been cast as shallow, narcissistic, untrustworthy, and morally bankrupt in character. These stereotypes are also driven by assumptions on bisexuals' (lack of) capacity for intimacy and their overt sexualisation. In activist contexts, bisexuals are often mistrusted as potential traitors to the lesbian and gay cause. They are seen as cop-outs or untrustworthy allies, who will 'desert' the struggle sooner or later. In some lesbian (feminist) contexts circulates the caution better to not get involved with a bi woman, since she is always destined to leave her lesbian partner for a man at one point in future (cf. Rust 1995, Ault 1996a, George 1993). The idea that bisexuals have the best of both worlds, are more in touch with their sexuality or have better chances for a date are the more benign versions of biphobic stereotypes.

Running up against stereotyped misrepresentation and overt forms of discrimination increases strain and stress levels in bi-identified people's lives. It may also complicate their relationship lives in the cases that bisexual people may be confronted with accusations, worries and resentments which stem from their partners investment in biphobic beliefs and assumptions. As we have seen, a range of biphobic stereotypes evolve around bisexuals' sexual selves and their feelings and behaviours in relationships. Research indicates that many (non-bisexual) people have reservations about getting involved with a bisexual person in the first place (Rust 1996a, Weinberg et al. 1994). This rejection or reluctance is fed by discourses which either question the moral integrity of bisexual people as such or represent relationships with bisexuals as doomed to fail. The pervasiveness of bi-negativity further adds to a social climate in which bisexual people find less support for their relationships. It is a widely shared insight in relationship and family studies that relationship maintenance is dependent on emotional and material support structures, a privilege which non-heterosexual relationship often find difficult to mobilise (Kurdek 1995).

Bisexuality and Kin Work

Kin work is a concept which originally emerged in the sociology of heterosexual family life in order to take account of the gendered division of labour invested in establishing and sustaining family ties. Research indicates that heterosexual women are more active than their male partners to build, foster and celebrate cross-household kin ties (Di Leonardo 1987). Creating and sustaining family ties is dependent on manifolds activities and communicative acts, including making phone calls, writing letters, organising holidays and social occasions, visiting other people, inviting friends and family members, preparing meals, selecting and purchasing gifts, doing favours and all the thought spent on making decisions on how to go about doing these things. Christopher Carrington (1999) has explored how this kind of kin work is undertaken and organised in non-heterosexual families. Carrington highlights the significance of class, profession, and 'race' or ethnicity in the ways in which same-sex partners engage in kin work. Anthropological and sociological research into queer family life has shown that gay men, lesbians and bisexuals have created family practices and family discourses which discard of the older perception that family is (exclusively) constituted through biology (reproduction) or legalised commitment (marriage). Queer people have engaged in the creation of what many call 'families of choice' which may be comprised of a particular blend of biological family ties, intimate partners, friends (individuals or family networks) and children (one's own or other family members') (Weston 1991, 1995). To a certain extent, heterosexual relationship cultures, too, have been drawn into family practices which transcend the logic of biology and state-sanctioned marriage. Researchers have described 'families of choice' as the 'new family practices' (Silva and Smart 1999) or as the prime example of 'postmodern families' (Stacey 1996). Carrington's (1999) research has been distinctive in highlighting that partners who are better off financially or whose professions' provide them some flexibility can do more kin work and thus frequently have more friends and larger family networks.

I am not so much interested in the division of labour between partners which has been the dominant perspective in the discussion on kin work. Rather, I would like to focus on the dimension of kin work which may stem from the indifference or hostility of some (potential) family members towards a same-sex partner. If kin work is about creating and maintaining family bonds than it is vital for friends and biological family to accept a same-sex partner as authentic family member in the first place. The life stories of many lesbians, gay men and bisexuals indicate that many have to cope with a great deal of hostility, if they reveal their sexual identities in their personal environments (Davies 1992). Biological family relationships are often particularly tricky. 'Coming out as lesbian, gay or bisexual to family can be traumatic, especially if relations with parents and siblings are difficult, or if they reject non-heterosexuality' (Weeks et al. 2001: 59). Even if the communication of queer identities has been 'normalised' to a certain extent in some cultural contexts (Seidman et al. 1999), many people still risk major ruptures in their close relationships, if not the loss of their family ties, if they decide to come out. The acknowledgement of this risk is at the heart of the normative stress on 'coming out' in LGBT or queer politics. For Black people, their biological families often provide an important bond in the struggle for survival in a racist society and family often provides a strong element within racial identification (Cohen 2001, Carrington 1999). For people who belong to groups subjected to racism it is not as easy to dismiss (biological) family ties, a position implicit in anti-family rhetoric of lesbian, gay male, bisexual and queer programmatic discourse common since the inception of 'gay liberation' (cf. GLF 1971/1995).

Making friends and family accept one's sexual identity and to embrace a same-sex partner in the face of out-right hostility is difficult and often depends on hurtful, persisting and subtle forms of kin work on the part of queer family members. Bisexuals are no exception here. Yet the fact that a bisexual person may have an other-sex partner in the future or may consider both same-sex and other-sex partners as family may trigger quite specific dynamics in conflictual kin work. Mariana Valverde (1985) has argued that in heterosexist society bisexuals are very likely to gain more recognition for and validation of their other-sex relationships than their same-sex relationships. Families may acknowledge a same-sex partner and consider him or her family but continue at the same time to invest in the hope that he or she may only be present for a transitory period. Of course, the same may be the case with regard to the partners of people who identify as gay or lesbian. Yet since hegemonic discourses construct bisexual identity foremost as unstable and transitory, such 'hopes' are much more likely to blossom in the case of bi-identified people struggling for the integration of their same-sex partners into their family. If bisexual people are non-monogamous or polyamorous and maintain relationships to both same-sex and other-sex partners, their friends and families may continue to ignore their same-sex partners or treat their partners on differential terms (Klesse 2007a). Legal marriage complicates this issue. Research indicates that many bi-identified people are legally married (Weinberg et al. 1994, George 1993). Valerie Lehr (1999) suggests that entering a civil marriage to a certain extent carries the potential to draw a person's same-sex relationships into the realm of the legitimate – at least within more libertarian cultural contexts. Current legislation in the UK prevents married bisexuals from marrying a second partner. Since there is no right for civil marriage between same-sex partners in current legal provisions, the only option would be a civil partnership in this case any way, a model perceived by many to be already illustrative of a second class status (Harding and Peel 2006, Clarke et al. 2006, Barker 2006). My own research into bisexual polyamorous bisexual relationships suggests that civil marriage is charged with an intense symbolism and carries the potential to demarcate the boundaries of family relationships. This means that bisexuals who are married may struggle hard to build families which integrate same-sex partners on equal terms. Yet the image of the marriage bond as determining a primary commitment may obstruct these efforts. To what extent the introduction of the UK Civil Partnership Act 2004 will alter these dynamics remains to be seen. It creates the basis of scenarios, in which a bisexual person first decides to enter a same-sex civil partnership and may than later wish to integrate a new partner with an other-sex person. This may alter the terms of negotiation and the (hetero)normative dynamics around it. Research indicates that the question of whether partners raise children together or not also has an impact on the construction of lesbian, gay and bisexual families, with child rearing partners being more likely to not consider friends as family (Carrington 1999). According to my knowledge, the dynamics around child rearing, different models of parenthood and discourses on kinship in polyamorous families has so far not yet been consistently explored (cf. Iantaffi 2006)

Bisexuality, Non-Monogamy and Polyamory

I have described the assumptions that bisexuals are promiscuous or by necessity non-monogamous as an element in the repertoire of bi-phobic representation. Many bisexual people commit themselves to monogamous partnerships. Yet bisexual relationship culture is rich in diversity (Rust 1996a, Hutchins 1996, Klesse 2007a). Research suggests a relatively high frequency of non-monogamous relationship arrangements among bisexual-identified men and women (cf. Blumstein and Schwartz 1983, Rust 1996a, Rodríguez Rust 2000c, Weinberg et al. 1994). Bisexual non-monogamies are extremely diverse. Non-monogamous relationships and families differ in terms of numbers of partners, degrees of closeness and commitment, legal relationship status, constellations of genders, social identities, household forms, parenting arrangements, etc. (Hutchins 1996, Pallotta-Chiarolli 1995, Paul 1997). People of all kinds of sexual identity and preference feel drawn towards non-monogamous lifestyles or a polyamorous relationship practice. It is impossible to generalise about a person's motivation for adopting a non-monogamous approach their relationship practice. The wish to be non-monogamous (or not to be in an exclusive couple relationship) may be fed by a variety of reasons which may include a mixture of emotional, sexual, political, economic, relationship internal or biographical factors. Yet my personal research indicates that at least some bi-identified people explain their wish to be non-monogamous with the bisexual (or pansexual) dimension of their desire.

Some research participants explained that sexual experience with people of one particular gender was so important to them that they would not be willing to give up on that option once they fell in love with a person of another gender. In particular women who had a primary involvement with women before they entered a long term relationships with a man found it impossible to give up on relationships with women, when they entered a partnership with a man. Others, often people who did not yet have a lot of same-sex experiences, did find it necessary to explore their same-sex desire and felt that monogamy would ultimately restrict their search for self-knowledge and self-realisation. The connections which some research participants established between their bisexual identity and their decision to be non-monogamous were often couched in highly personal language. Yet it is not difficult to see how political values come into the equation as well. These may involve a feminist endorsement of female sexual autonomy or close intimate bonds between women (Gregory 1983, Klesse 2009), a rejection of hegemonic monosexuality (Rodriguez Rust 2000c) or a commitment to a sex-positive queer culture (Haritaworn et al. 2006). The above mentioned positions are examples from the life histories and relationship narratives of a small number of research participants. I do not suggest that they are representative of the orientations and feelings of polyamorous bisexuals. I do not claim this to be an exhaustive analysis of the subject matter either. While a bisexual and a polyamorous identity may intersect for some people, this is not necessarily always the case. The coincidence of these identities may be also be accidental. Some research participants in my study did stress the distinctiveness and independence of their investment in bisexual and polyamorous identities (Klesse 2007a). Some may opt to be non-monogamous for reasons other than their bisexuality, for example, if they wish to express or explore dimensions of their eroticism which their current partner does not wish to share (such as for example certain BDSM practices) (cf. Langdridge and Barker 2007).

Bisexuals who wish to be non-monogamous and polyamorous frequently have to negotiate a range of issues in their relationships. Monogamy is a value deeply engrained in dominant culture and provides the ground for far-reaching moral judgements. People in non-monogamous and polyamorous relationships face serious stigmatisation. They are usually cast as immoral, narcissistic, immature and sex-crazed. These kind of allegation can be aggravated by racist, classist and sexist stereotypical ascriptions (Klesse 2005). Moreover, the monogamous couple is construed as the only route to a successful relationship life. Even among the most liberal and well-meaning observers, multiple partner constellation are usually considered to be rather daring experiments which do not carry any realistic chance to survive in the long-term. Thus, polyamorous partners are quite likely to find themselves confronted with a less than encouraging, if not out-right hostile, environment. If polyamorous bisexuals raise children social stigmatisation intensifies. Normative discourses on parenthood and in particular motherhood provide the fodder for accusations of irresponsibility (cf. Iantaffi 2006). The absence of intelligible models or even a commonly understood language for multiple relationships render it difficult and an odd experience for polyamorous partners to explain their relationships to people who are not familiar with polyamorous practice (Ritchie and Barker 2006, Barker 2005).

Yet there may also be relationship internal conflicts. Problems will most certainly arise, if the current partner of a polyamorous-inclined person feels uncomfortable with a non-monogamous arrangement (Weitzman 2006). These problems may come up at an early stage once the issue of opening or expanding the relationship has been brought up. Yet they may also emerge at later point, if a partner's comfort with or interest in a polyamorous or non-monogamous relationship arrangement is fading. There may also be conflicts about the terms or the kind of an arrangement around non-monogamy. Over recent years a growing set of self-help manuals emerged, which provide advise on how partners may proceed to find solutions in the case of such conflicts.[4] Most of these texts take a fairly optimistic stance on how the problems can be settled and do not consider how power imbalances between partners may complicate a satisfying consensus-based solution (Noël 2006). For people who seek therapy and counselling in a situation of a relationship conflict around non-monogamy it is vital to have the opportunity work with a person who is not judgemental and has not issues with the actual diversity of sexual and intimate practices among bisexual people (Weitzman 2006).

Conclusion

Dominant understandings of sexuality assume that people are either straight or homosexual. Many do still not consider bisexuality to represent an authentic and mature sexual identity. This has a variety of consequences in the lives of people who identify as bisexual or who do not conceal the fact that they do not limit their erotic attention to one gender only. Common anti-bi sentiments complicate bisexual identification, bisexual coming or being 'out' and the maintenance of bisexual intimacies. Bisexual behaviours may be disapproved of, ignored, played down in significance, interpreted as transitory confusions or subsumed to essentialist identity narratives. The bisexuality of bisexuals may disappear in the eyes and memories of their environment, if they are in monogamous relationships. Their bisexuality is all too often seen as scandalous if they want to act on it or if they are in non-monogamous or multiple relationships. Bisexuality is read as a sign of instability. Bisexual identities are assumed to disappear in the process of

---

4   The most prominent manual of this case is probably *The Ethical Slut* by Dossie Easton and Catherine Liszt (1997) which many polyamorous people consider to be the 'bible of polyamory'. For a critical overview on this literature, see Petrella 2007, Noël 2006, and Klesse 2007b.

maturation and growing self-knowledge. Relationships with a bisexual partner are construed as risky and short-living. Bisexuals who maintain non-monogamous relationships are assumed to fulfil the prophecy of powerful stereotypes. Their relationships and families are pathologised and diagnosed to fail. The awkward role of bisexuality in a signification of sexual difference based on a foundational duality expels from the realm of intelligible intimacy into the virtual spaces of the un-real. This inevitably creates problems in the intimate lives for bisexual-identified people. Therapists and counsellors who work with bisexual clients thus need a nuanced understanding of how the contradictory discourses around bisexuality feed into a repertoire of anti-bisexual sentiments. An awareness of the manifold manifestations of biphobia is the precondition for supporting bisexual people effectively and in a professional and person affirmative manner.

References

Adam, B.D. (1998), 'Theorizing homophobia', *Sexualities*, 1(4), pp. 387–404.

Angelides, S. (2000), *A History of Bisexuality*, Chicago: The University of Chicago Press.

Atkins, D. (ed.) (2002), *Bisexual Women in the Twenty-First Century*, New York: Harrington Park Press.

Ault, A. (1996a), 'Hegemonic discourse in an oppositional community: Lesbian feminist stigmatization of bisexual women', in B. Beemyn and M. Eliason (eds), *Queer Studies. A Lesbian, Gay, Bisexual, and Transgender Anthology*, London: New York University Press, pp. 204–216.

Ault, A. (1999), 'Ambiguous identity in an unambiguous sex/gender structure: The case of bisexual women', in M. Storr (ed.), *Bisexuality: A Critical Reader*, London: Routledge, pp. 167–186.

Barker, M. (2005), 'This is my partner, and this is my ... partner's partner: Constructing a polyamorous identity in a monogamous world', *Journal of Constructivist Psychology*, 18(1), pp. 75–88.

Barker, N. (2004), 'For better or worse? The Civil Partnership Bill 2004', *Journal of Social Welfare and Family Law*, 26(3), pp. 313–324.

Barker, N. (2006), 'Sex and the Civil Partnership Act: The future of (non) conjugality?', *Feminist Legal Studies*, 14(2), August 2006, pp. 241–259.

Bell, D. (1994), 'Bisexuality: A place on the margins', in S. Whittle (ed.), *The Margins of the City*, Aldershot: Ashgate.

Bell, D. and Binnie, J. (2000), *The Sexual Citizen. Queer Politics and Beyond*, Cambridge: Polity Press.

Berlant, L. and Warner, M. (1998), 'Sex in public', *Critical Inquiry*, No. 24, pp. 547–566.

Bi Academic Intervention (ed.) (1997), *The Bisexual Imaginary. Representation, Identity and Desire*, London: Cassell.

Binnie J. (1997), 'Invisible Europeans: Sexual citizenship in the New Europe', *Environment and Planning A*, 29, 182–199.

Blumstein, P. and Schwartz, P. (1983), *American Couples*, New York: William Morrow.

Bower, J., Gurevich, M. and Mathieson, C. (2002), '(Con)tested identities: Bisexual women reorient sexuality', in D. Atkins (ed.), *Bisexual Women in the Twenty-First Century*, New York: Harrington Park Press, pp. 25–52.

Bristow, J. (1997), *Sexuality*, London: Routledge.

Butler, J. (1990), *Gender Trouble. Feminism and the Subversion of Identity*, London: Routledge.

Butler, J. (1993), *Bodies that Matter: On the Discursive Limits of 'Sex'*, London: Routledge.

Califia, P. (1997), *Sex Changes. The Politics of Transgenderism*, San Francisco: Cleis Press.

Carrington, C. (1999), *No Place Like Home. Relationships and Family Life among Lesbians and Gay Men*, London: University of Chicago Press.

Clarke, V., Burgoyne, C. and Burns, M. (2006), 'Just a piece of paper? A qualitative exploration of same-sex couples multiple conceptions of civil partnership and marriage', *Lesbian and Gay Psychology Review*, 7(2), July 2006 (Special Feature: Same-Sex Marriage), pp. 14–161.

Cohen, C.J. (2001), 'Punks, bulldaggers, and welfare queens', in M. Blasius (ed.), *Sexual Identities, Queer Politics*, Oxford: Princeton University Press, pp. 200–227.

Cossman, B. (2007), *Sexual Citizens. The Legal and Cultural Regulations of Sex and Belonging*, Stanford, CA: Stanford University Press.

Davies, D. (2003), 'Homophobia and heterosexism', in D. Davies and C. Neal (ed.), *Pink Therapy. A Guide for Counsellors and Therapists Working with Lesbians, Gay and Bisexual Clients*, Maidenhead: Open University Press, pp. 41–65.

Davies, D. (2003), 'Towards a model of affirmative therapy', in D. Davies and C. Neal (ed.), *Pink Therapy. A Guide for Counsellors and Therapists Working with Lesbians, Gay and Bisexual Clients*, Maidenhead: Open University Press, pp. 24–40.

Davies, D. and Neal, C. (eds) (2000), *Therapeutic Perspectives on Working with Lesbian, Gay and Bisexual Clients*, Buckingham: Open University Press.

Davies, D. and Neal, C. (eds) (2003), *Pink Therapy. A Guide for Counsellors and Therapists Working with Lesbians, Gay and Bisexual Clients*, Maidenhead: Open University Press.

Davies, P. (1992), 'The role of coming out among gay men' in K. Plummer (ed.), *Modern Homosexualities. Fragments of Lesbian and Gay Experience*, London: Routledge.

Di Leonardo, M. (1987), 'The female world of cards and holidays: Women, families, and the work of kinship', *Signs 12* (Summer), 440–452.

Easton, D. and Liszt, C.A. (1997), *The Ethical Slut*, San Francisco: Greenery Press.

Ellis, M. (1999), 'En-gendering a race perspective', BCN 34 (February 1999) <http://bcn.bi.org/issue34/genderrace.html> (accessed: 29/09/04).

Evans, D.T. (1993), *Sexual Citizenship: The Material Construction of Sexualities*, London: Routledge.

Gamson, J. (1998), *Freaks Talk Back*, Chicago: University of Chicago Press.

George, S. (1993), *Women and Bisexuality*, London: Scarlet Press.

GLF (1971/1995), 'GLF manifesto', in L. Power (ed.), *No Bath But Plenty of Bubbles. An Oral History of the Gay Liberation Front 1970–1973*, London: Cassell.

Gorna, R. (1996), *Vamps, Virgins and Victims: How Can Women Fight AIDS?* London: Cassell.

Gregory, D. (1983), 'From where I stand: A case for feminist bisexuality', in S. Cartledge and J. Ryan (eds), *Sex and Love. New Thoughts and Old Contradictions*, London: The Women's Press Ltd., pp. 141–156.

Hall, S. (1992), 'The question of cultural identity', in S. Hall, D. Held and T. McGrew (eds), *Modernity and its Futures* (in association with the Open University), London: Polity Press, pp. 274–316.

Hall, S. (1996), 'Introduction: Who needs "identity"', in S. Hall and P. du Gay (eds), *Questions of Cultural Identity*, London: Sage, pp. 1–17.

Harding, R. and Peel, L. (2006), '"We do?" International perspectives on equality, legality and same-sex relationships', *Lesbian and Gay Psychology Review*, 7(2), July 2006 (Special Feature: Same-Sex Marriage), pp. 141–161.

Haritaworn, J., Lin C.J. and Klesse, C. (2006), 'Poly/logue: A critical introduction to polyamory', *Sexualities*, 9(5), December 2006 (Special Issue on Polyamory), pp. 515–529.

Heaphy, B. (2007), 'Same-sex marriage/civil unions', in G. Ritzer (ed.), *The Blackwell Encyclopaedia of Sociology Vol. VIII*, Oxford: Blackwell Publishers, pp. 3995–3998.

Hemmings, C. (2002), *Bisexual Spaces. Geography of Sexuality and Gender*, London: Routledge.

Hennessy, R. (1995), 'Queer visibility in commodity culture', in L. Nicholson and S. Seidman (eds), *Social Postmodernism: Beyond Identity Politics*, Cambridge: Cambridge University Press.

Hodges, A. and Hutter, D. (1974), *With Downcast Gays*, London: Pomegranate Press, GLF Pamphlet.

Howarth, D. (2000), *Discourse*, Buckingham: Open University Press.

Howarth, D. and Stavrakakis, Y. (2000), 'Introducing discourse theory and political analysis', in D. Howarth and A.J. Norval and Y. Stavrakakis (eds), *Discourse Theory and Political Analysis. Identities, Hegemonies and Social Change*, Manchester and New York: Manchester University Press, pp. 1–23.

Hodges, A. and Hutter, D. (1974), *With Downcast Gays*, London: Pomegranate Press (GLF Pamphlet).

Hutchins, L. (1996), 'Bisexuality: Politics and community', in B.A. Firestein (ed.), *Bisexuality. The Psychology and Politics of an Invisible Minority*, London: Sage Hutchinson.

Iantaffi, A. (2006), 'Polyamory and parenting: Some personal reflections', *Lesbian and Gay Psychology Review*, 7(1), pp. 70–72.

Island, D and Letellier, P. (1992), *Men Who Beat the Men Who Love Them*, New York: Harrington Park Press.

Jamieson, L. (1998), *Intimacy: Personal Relationships in Modern Societies*, Cambridge: Polity.

Jordan, J. (1996), 'A new politics of sexuality', in S. Rose, C. Stevens et al. (eds), *Off Pink Collective Bisexual Horizons: Politics, Histories, Lives*, London: Lawrence and Wishart, pp. 11–15.

Klesse, C. (2005), 'Bisexual women, non-monogamy, and differentialist anti-promiscuity discourses', *Sexualities*, 8(4), pp. 445–464.

Klesse, C. (2007a), *The Spectre of Promiscuity: Gay Male and Bisexual Non-Monogamies and Polyamories*, Aldershot: Ashgate.

Klesse, C. (2007b), '"How to be a happy homosexual?!" Non-monogamy and governmentality in relationship manuals for gay men in the 1980s and 1990s', *The Sociological Review*, 55(3), August, pp. 571–591.

Klesse, C. (2009) 'Paradoxes in gender relations: [Post] feminism and bisexual non-monogamy and polyamory', in M. Barker and D. Langdridge (eds), *Understanding Non-Monogamies*, London: Routledge.

Kofman, E., Phizacklea, A., Raghuram, P. and Sales, R. (2000), *Gender and International Migration in Europe. Employment, Welfare and Politics*, London: Routledge.

Kurdek, L.A. (1995), 'Lesbian and gay couples', in R.D. Augelli and C.J. Patterson (eds), *Lesbian, Gay and Bisexual Identities over the Lifespan. Psychological Perspectives*, New York and Oxford: Oxford University Press, pp. 243–261.

Laclau, E. (1990), *New Reflections on the Revolution of Our Time*, London: Verso.

Langdridge, D. and Barker, M. (eds) (2007), *Safe, Sane and Consensual: Contemporary Perspectives on Sadomasochism*, Basingstoke: Palgrave Macmillan.

Lehr, V. (1999), *Queer Family Values. Debunking the Myth of the Nuclear Family*, Philadelphia: Temple University Press.

Leventhal, B. and Lundy, S.E. (eds) (1999), *Same-Sex Domestic Violence: Strategies for Change*, London: Sage.

Mercer, K. and Isaac, J. (1988), 'Race, sexual politics and black masculinity. A dossier', in J. Rutherford and R. Chapman (eds), *Unwrapping Masculinity*, London: Lawrence and Wishart, pp. 97–130.

Monk, D. (2009), 'Engaging with the law: Cause to celebrate and time to question', paper presented at the UCU LGBT History Conference, 29 February 2009, Manchester Metropolitan University, UK.

Moon, L. (ed.) (2008), *Feeling Queer or Queer Feelings. Radical Approaches to Counselling Sex, Sexualities and Genders*, London: Routledge.

Neal, C. and Davis, D. (eds) (2000a), *Issues in Therapy with Lesbian, Gay, Bisexual and Transgender Clients*, Buckingham: Open University Press.

Neal, C. and Davis, D. (2000b), 'Introduction', in C. Neal and D. Davis (eds), *Issues in Therapy with lesbian, Gay, Bisexual and Transgender Clients*, Buckingham: Open University Press, pp. 1–6.

Nestle, J. Howell, C. and Wilkins R. (eds) (2002), *GenderQueer: Voices from beyond the Sexual Binary*, Los Angeles, CA: Alyson Books.

Noël, M.J. (2006), 'Progressive polyamory: Conisdering issues of diversity', *Sexualities*, 9(5), December 2006, pp. 602–619.

Ochs, R. (1996), 'Biphobia: It goes more than two ways', in B.A. Firestein (ed.), *Bisexuality. The Psychology and Politics of an Invisible Minority*, London: Sage, pp. 217–239.

Oxley, E. and Lucius, C.A. (2000), 'Looking both ways: Bisexuality and therapy', in C. Neal and D. Davis (eds), *Issues in Therapy with Lesbian, Gay, Bisexual and Transgender Clients*, Buckingham: Open University Press, pp. 115–127.

Pallotta-Chiarolli, M. (1995), 'Choosing not to choose: Beyond monogamy, beyond duality', in K. Lano and C. Parry (eds), *Breaking the Barriers to Desire. New Approaches to Multiple Relationships*, Nottingham: Five Leaves Publications, pp. 41–67.

Paul, J.P. (1997), 'Bisexuality: Exploring/exploding the binaries', in R.C. Savin-Williams and K.M. Cohen (eds), *The Lives of Lesbians, Gays and Bisexuals. Children to Adults*, Orlando, FL: Harcourt Brace and Company, pp. 436–461.

Peplau, L.A., Venigas, R.C. and Miller Campbell, S. (1997), 'Gay and lesbian relationships', in R.C. Savin-Williams and K.M. Cohen (eds), *The Lives of Lesbians, Gays and Bisexuals. Children to Adults*, Orlando, FL: Harcourt Brace and Company, pp. 250–273.

Petrella, S. (2007), 'Ethical sluts and closet polyamorists: Dissident eroticism, abject subjects and the normative cycle in self-help books on free love', in N. Rumens and A. Cervantes-Carson (eds), *The Sexual Politics of Desire and Belonging*, Rodopi: Tijnmuiden, pp. 151–170.

Queen, C. (1996), 'Sexual diversity and bisexual identity', in N. Tucker (with R. Kaplan) (eds), *Bisexual Politics. Theories, Queries and Visions*, Binghamton: Harrington Park Press, pp. 151–160.

Richardson, D. (2000), *Rethinking Sexuality*, London: Sage.

Ritchie, A. and Barker, M. (2006), '"There aren't words for what we do of how we fell so we have to make them up": Constructing polyamorous languages in a culture of compulsory monogamy', *Sexualities*, 9(5), December 2006, pp. 584–601.

Rodríguez Rust, P.C. (2000a), 'Alternatives to binary sexuality: Modelling bisexuality', in P.C. Rodríguez Rust (ed.), *Bisexuality in the United States. A Social Science Reader*, New York: Columbia University Press, pp. 33–54.

Rodríguez Rust, P.C. (2000b), 'Heterosexual gays, heterosexual lesbians and homosexual straights', in P.C. Rodríguez Rust (ed.), *Bisexuality in the United*

States. A Social Science Reader, New York: Columbia University Press, pp. 279–306.

Rodríguez Rust, P.C. (2000c), 'The biology, psychology, sociology and sexuality of bisexuality', in P.C. Rodríguez Rust (ed.), *Bisexuality in the United States. A Social Science Reader*, New York: Columbia University Press, pp. 403–470.

Rust, P.C. (1995), *Bisexuality and the Challenge to Lesbian Politics. Sex, Loyalty and Revolution*, New York: New York University Press.

Rust, P.C. (1996a), 'Monogamy and polyamory: Relationship issues for bisexuals', in B.A. Firestein (ed.), *Bisexuality. The Psychology and Politics of an Invisible Minority*, London: Sage, pp. 127–148.

Rust, P.C. (1996b), 'Sexual identities: The struggle for self-description in a changing sexual landscape', in B. Beemyn and M. Eliason (eds), *Queer Studies. A Lesbian, Gay, Bisexual and Transgender Anthology*, New York: New York University Press.

Sedgwick, E.K. (1993), 'How to bring your kids up gay', in M. Warner (ed.), *Fear of a Queer Planet. Queer Politics and Social Theory*, Minneapolis: University of Minnesota Press, 69–81.

Seidman, S., Meeks, C. and Traschen, F. (1999), 'Beyond the closet? The changing social meaning of homosexuality in the United States', *Sexualities*, 2(1), February, pp. 9–34.

Silva, E.B. and Smart, C.B. (1999b), 'The "new" practices of family life', in E.B. Silva and C. Smart (eds), *The New Family?* London: Sage, pp. 1–12.

Simmons, T. (2007), 'Sexuality and immigration: UK family reunion policy and the regulation of sexual citizens in the European Union', *Political Geography*, 27(2), February 2008, pp. 213–230.

Solomos, J. (2003), *Race and Racism in Britain* (3rd Edition), Basingstoke: Palgrave Macmillan.

Stacey, J. (1996), *In the Name of the Family. Rethinking Family Values in the Postmodern Age*, Boston: Beacon Press.

Stein, A. (1997), *Sex and Sensibility. Stories of a Lesbian Generation*, Berkeley: University of California Press.

Storr, M. (1997), 'The sexual reproduction of "race": Bisexuality, history and racialisation', in Bi Academic Intervention (ed.), *The Bisexual Imaginary*, London: Cassell, pp. 73–88.

Stychin, C. (2003), *Governing Sexuality. The Changing Politics of Citizenship and Law Reform*, Oxford: Hart.

Udis-Kessler, A. (1996b), 'Challenging the stereotypes', in Off Pink Collective (ed.), *Bisexual Horizons. Politics, Histories, Lives*, London: Lawrence and Wishart.

Valverde, M. (1985), *Sex, Power and Pleasure*, Toronto, Ontario: The Women's Press.

Weeks, J. (1990), *Coming-Out: Homosexual Politics in Britain from the Nineteenth Century to the Present* (2nd Edition), London: Quartet.

Weeks, J., Donovan, C. and Heaphy, B. (1996), *Families of Choice: Patterns of Non-Heterosexual Relationships. A Literature Review*, Social Science Research Papers No. 2, School of Education and Social Science, Southbank University, London.

Weeks, J., Heaphy, B., Donovan, C. (2001), *Same-Sex Intimacies. Families of Choice and Other Life Experiments*, London: Routledge.

Weinberg, M.S., Williams, C.J. and Pryor D.W. (1994), *Dual Attraction. Understanding Bisexuality*, New York and Oxford: Oxford University Press.

Weitzman, G. (2006), 'What psychology professionals should know about polyamory', *Journal of Bisexuality*, 6(1/2), pp. 137–164.

Weston, K. (1991), *Families We Choose: Lesbians, Gays, Kinship*, New York: Columbia University Press.

Whittle, S. (2002), *Respect and Equality. Transsexual and Transgender Rights*, London: Cavendish Publishing.

Wintemute, R. and Andenœs, M. (eds) (2001), *Legal Recognition of Same-Sex Partnerships: A Study of National, European and International Law*, Oxford and Portland, Oregon: Hart.

Ytterberg, H. (2008), 'So why can't they just be satisfied with civil partnership? Does marriage matter, or is it all about semantics?', seminar paper presented at the School of Law, Manchester Metropolitan University, 17 December 2008.

Zinik, G. (1985), 'Identity conflict or adaptive flexibility? Bisexuality reconsidered', in F. Klein and T. Wolf (eds), *Bisexualities*, London: The Haworth Press, pp. 7–20.

Chapter 8

Multiple Identities, Multiple Realities: Lesbian, Gay and Queer Lives in the North East of England

Mark Casey

Through drawing upon research undertaken in the city of Newcastle upon Tyne this chapter will theorise the intersection of experiences in queer scene spaces and the lesbian and gay home with mental health concerns. The multiple identities lesbians and gay men possess or make claims to and how they intersect with spatial experiences within the North East of England will be the key focus. The complexity offered through late modernity and the identities it supports has the consequence that identities such as lesbian, gay or queer[1] can no longer be theorised as standing separate to other identities. The chapter will theorise the intersecting of sexual identity with gender, age, disability and socio-economic class, which in turn intersect with spatial inclusions/exclusions. In so doing the chapter wishes to draw attention for those working in the mental health profession to the diverse material realities of lesbians and gay men, and the consequential multiple mental health needs of this population. The chapter will conclude through addressing the unique mental health needs of lesbians and gay men and how these are impacted by both societal homophobia but also pressures from within the wider lesbian and gay community.

Opinions upon homosexuality and/or gay male and lesbian sexuality have changed significantly since the 1970s within the wider public and those working within the mental health profession. Few topics have proven more controversial in the field of psychiatry, with homosexuality being classified as a mental disorder and/or deviation since the late nineteenth century and for much of the

---

1   Queer evolved as a political protest and post-identity movement in the early 1990s with the advent of Queer Nation and ACT UP. Political groups who wished to move beyond the limits of lesbian, gay *and* heterosexual identities embraced the term and project. Such political actions seemed to fail with the eventual success of assimilationist politics (see Bawer, 1994). Queer is now more commonly linked and theorised within the academy under Queer Theory (see Richardson et al., 2006). Although queer is drawn upon within this chapter to refer to non-normative sexual identities and practices, the terms and identities of lesbian and gay are used throughout due to the claiming and use of these by the research participants referred to in this chapter.

twentieth century (Bailey, 1999; Sandfort, 2001). As Nye (1999) reminds us, it was the medical profession who named, classified and problematised the modern homosexual. In the US and Western Europe during the 1960s and 1970s, the feminist and gay rights movements worked hard to change the negative views on homosexuality which positioned it as a sickness and the inferior *other* to heterosexuality. For example, in the first edition of the 1952 *Diagnostic and Statistical Manual of Mental Disorders* 'homosexuality' was characterised as a sociopathic personality disorder. Although the 1968 revised edition was milder in tone, heterosexuality was still positioned as the norm with homosexuality classified as a problematic deviation from this (Campos and Goldfried, 2001, 610). Writing in 1969, Sandor Rado argued that the only non-pathological outcome for a person's sexual orientation was heterosexuality. Equally for Ovesey (1969), a neutral psychoanalytical stance towards homosexuality was unacceptable. Ovesey argued that for the homosexual to overcome his homosexuality he would have to engage in actual heterosexual sex acts which would act as a 'cure', (Ovesey gave no thought to lesbian sexuality) (Halpert, 2000, 20). As such, these problematic classifications were discussed and moved from theory into practice. The gay rights movement rejected negative medicalised models of 'the homosexual' and moved to claim the right to name their own identity as gay men and lesbians. Through the naming and claiming of their own sexual identity, gay men and lesbians were now denying negative medical authority over their sexual identities and practice (Engel, 2002, 38). As Cruikshank (1992, 3) has argued, 'homosexuals became gay when they rejected the notion that they were sick or sinful …', he goes onto claim that 'above all gay was a name chosen by the group itself, as sign of its refusal to be named, judged or controlled by the dominant majority' (1992, 9). In response to growing cultural and political changes in the US, in 1973 the American Psychiatric Association (ASA) removed homosexuality from its list of mental health illnesses (Sandfort et al., 2001). After the ASA's decision, Watters (1986) noted a significant increase during the early 1980s in research articles published within the mental health arena that addressed homosexuals positively. In the UK, clinicians during this period began to adopt models of treatment for lesbians and gay men focused upon improving their sexual identities and lives, rather than trying to change them. This shift can be seen as initially legislative, reflecting that therapists are not necessarily separate from the social world and the norms and stigma it posses. Mental health practitioners were increasingly becoming aware of the mental health issues of their lesbian and gay clients that were (and still are) unique given the stressors related to same-sex sexual identities, such as victimisation, harassment, fear of rejection from family and friends and the wider culture of homophobia (Berg et al., 2008; Glazer et al., 2008). In 1992 the World Health Organisation (WHO) declassified homosexuality as a mental health illness (Pett, 2000, 55), although this is a stance that many countries have not adopted, such as Iran, China and Poland.

More recent research on mental health[2] and wellbeing (see Diaz et al., 2001; Koh and Ross, 2006; Sandfort et al., 2006; Berg et al., 2008) has challenged the accepted binary that once privileged heterosexuality as the norm, and homosexuality as the problematic 'other'. Such developments do not completely remove homophobic[3] beliefs and opinions which can be present within therapists' values. For example, for those practitioners who had been educated in a time when homosexuality was positioned as a disorder, new ways of approaching the gay or lesbian client may not necessarily be welcomed. As Kaufman et al. (1997) discussed, views which could be deemed to be homophobic were found to be present in some therapists' values and in gay men's and lesbians' experiences of therapy. In reflecting on his own heterosexuality, Miller (2008, 382) argues that for heterosexual therapists their own sexuality inevitably plays a role in their experiences and interactions with patients. Even if therapists do not understand themselves as homophobic, they may still have values that position heterosexuality as the given norm. Bailey (1999, 884) suggests, somewhat problematically, that gay men may suffer more mental health problems than heterosexual men due to their shared mental health traits with heterosexual women. It can be argued that such an approach continues to position gay men against and inferior to, 'real' heterosexual men. Work which claimed to have found evidence of biological foundations to gay male sexuality was widely publicised and well received by (certain) sections of the scientific, medical and gay communities in the 1990s (see Ingraham, 2002). Simon Le Vay (1991) claimed that gay men's brains were different to those of other men, while Dean Hammer (1993) believed that there was a (potential) difference in the genes of gay men. However this work presents a number of flaws – from the research populations accessed, to the way analysis was undertaken, which problematises the strength of any claims made (see Brokey, 2000). When adopting such research in working with lesbian or gay clients, practitioners should question what are the motives behind this research and examine both the costs and value of drawing upon these research findings for clients. Sorensen and Roberts through their focus upon lesbians have commented that there is a continued heterosexual bias in research on women's physical and mental health. For example, they argue 'the bulk of research about women's health presumes all women to be heterosexual and has thus focused on gynaecological and reproductive concerns' (1997, 46). However, Liddle (1999) argues that better training of mental health practitioners

---

2   Symptoms of poor mental heath for the purpose of this chapter are understood as 'common psychiatric disorders' (such as depression, anxiety, substance abuse) and suicidal behaviours (for a further discussion see Fergusson et al., 1999).

3   In drawing upon the work of Diaz et al. (2001) understandings and experiences of homophobia can be engaged with. In their research on gay men and mental health, Diaz et al. used 11 items to measure experiences of homophobia which encompasses not only the threat and use of homophobic violence and abuse against a person, but includes the privileging of heterosexuality and the need to perform a heterosexual identity to avoid violence and shame in both public and private sites (2001, 928).

and wider societal changes have been found to be beneficial for lesbians and gay men's experiences with therapists. In citing her own research, Liddle showcases how ratings by lesbians and gay men of heterosexual therapists have shifted from 'not at all helpful' in the late 1980s to 'very helpful' by the mid-1990s.[4]

At one time homosexuality was treated as a serious mental disorder, but practitioners today are expected to understand lesbian and gay male identity and sexual practice as having equal value to that of heterosexuality. However we must be careful not to equate this with in-depth knowledge of or skill with working with lesbians and gay men. As the work of Moon (2007) has shown, the codes of ethics for mental health practitioners suggest non-discriminatory practice – however there is often little effort to adhere to this. For example, training that incorporates sexuality may have the subject 'added onto' other issues such as 'social contexts' or 'difference and diversity'. Moon's (2007) research suggests that in seven years of training the maximum focus most therapists will have about sex, sexuality or gender is only 16 hours, with courses continuing to be embedded with heteronormative bias. Avery et al. (2001, 990) suggests that little is still known about the specificities of treatment needs of lesbians and gay men with mental health issues. However, Neal and Davis (2000, 1) suggest that knowledge in this field is growing significantly with therapists working with lesbians and gay men being encouraged to strive to have a good level of self-awareness and comfort with all sexualities. Maylon (1982, 69) describes gay affirmative therapy as challenging the view that homosexual desire and orientations are pathological and regards homophobia rather than homosexuality as a major pathological factor. Much recent research on lesbians and gay men's mental health supports these claims (Koh and Ross, 2006; Sandfort et al., 2006; McDowell and Serovich, 2007), with Diaz et al. (2001, 931) arguing that poor mental health indicators, such as low self-esteem amongst gay men, must be addressed in programmes designed to improve gay men's mental well-being. Research by both Liddle (1999) and Koh and Ross (2006) have found similar findings with lesbian clients. For both Isay (1989) and Davies (1996) a 'core condition' of respect is needed for the client's sexual identity for personal integrity, lifestyle and culture, together with respectful attitudes on the therapist's own part. For Berg et al. (2008) therapists working with lesbians and gay men need to have an openness and awareness of the needs of their clients, where problems associated with being gay or lesbian are not due to these being problematic sexual identities, but due to wider societal homophobia:

> Understanding the mental health needs of gay and bisexual individuals is important because of the unique stressors related to one's same sex sexual

---

4   Through the work of those such as Dr Miller in Northern Ireland and his 'curing' of gay men and lesbians of their 'problematic' homosexuality, lesbians and gay men are reminded of the continued privileging of heterosexuality and problematising of homosexuality by those in the medical profession (see BBC News Online, 07.08.08).

orientation such as victimization, harassment, fear of rejection from friends and family, as well as possible discrimination. (2008, 294)

Since the 1990s (e.g. Garnets and Kimmel, 1993; Adam, 2000; Halpert, 2000; Avery, 2001; Koh and Ross, 2006; Sandfort et al., 2006) a shift has been present in mental health practice where sexual identity itself is not pathologised as the sole factor in seeking out professional help. As Davison (2001, 696) has argued, many of the issues presented by gay men are the same for which heterosexual men will seek help; performance anxiety, depression, substance abuse, social phobias and suicidal behaviours. Sorenson and Roberts (1997) through their focus on lesbian users of mental health services found that many lesbians who had mental health concerns did so, not necessarily because of their sexuality, but because of everyday stressors. Lesbians within their research cited work difficulties, money worries, relationships problems and substance abuse – issues presented were not dissimilar to the concerns of many heterosexual clients (1997, 37). However, such research should not be understood as minimising the potential impact of sexual identity upon the mental health needs of lesbians and gay men. Davison (2001) goes onto strongly suggest that continued discrimination, hostility and violence toward gay men (and lesbians) within most societies has serious consequences for the mental health of these groups. Abelson et al. (2006) and Berg et al. (2008) support Davison: in both their studies sexual identity was found to be an indicator of suicide risk. Their findings suggested that gay men did in fact have a higher risk of suicide compared with heterosexual men. Research by both Fergusson et al. (1999) and Sandfort et al. (2001, 2006) has unearthed similar findings, although such a link to suicide was not due to some biological link from being a gay man. The higher incidence of suicide attempts and actual deaths from suicide amongst gay men must be attributed to greater pressures upon gay men from heterosexual hatred and the violence and stigma this can bring. Abelson et al. (2006) in drawing upon Durkheim's theory of suicide, reflect that widespread homophobia[5] provides a framework for understanding a higher incidence of suicidal behaviours amongst gay men (and lesbians).

The development of a gay male or lesbian identity through the act of 'coming out' is the centre of much work on lesbian and gay sexuality, where identity development and the acquisition of a stable and enjoyable sexual identity is to be experienced (see Kort, 2008). These approaches typically propose a number of stage theories laying out a process of individual transition toward self-acceptance (see Adam, 2000, 325). A study by Koh and Ross (2006) on lesbian, bisexual and heterosexual women found that the level of 'outness' experienced by a lesbian was directly linked to good mental health. Sorenson and Roberts (1997, 47) echo

---

5   Although homophobia is often used to describe violence, hate and verbal attacks against lesbians and gay men, it should also be understood as including heterosexual bias and heteronormative assumptions often present in 'tolerant' and 'accepting' environments (see Casey, 2002).

these findings, suggesting that incidences of suicide amongst lesbians decrease as they age and experience a successful 'coming out' and acceptance of their sexual identity. Similar findings have been found to be true for gay men (Kort, 2008). Although 'coming out' may be a key goal for many lesbians and gay men, we must be careful not to map expected linear 'developmental stages' of sexual identity development onto all lesbians and gay men. The suggestion that all lesbians and gay men must go through multiple stages of coming out, acceptance, finding a partner and so on, ignores diversity in life goals, experiences and lived realities. Developmental stages may be useful for some lesbians and gay men, but a 'one size fits all' approach to lesbian and gay sexual identities can be limiting and problematic.

When gay men and lesbians have access to wide social networks of other gay men, lesbians and/or accepting heterosexuals and reject negative stereotypes provided by society, they are able to produce and nurture a positive identity and self-concept. But as Ueno (2005) reminds us, support for younger gay men is often lacking. Unlike heterosexual teen's that can often turn to their parents for support concerning relationship and identity issues, for lesbian and gay teen's parent's attitudes towards their child's sexual identity will vary considerably. The response of parent's, positive or negative, will assert a strong influence on adolescent's psychological state (2005, 259). Support for lesbian and gay youth from peers and family when coming out, is central to good mental well-being as well as an embracing of their own sexual identity (Casey, 2002). For those gay men who can access gay male sub-cultures and social groups they may be able to foster a group identity, in which role models are provided and feelings of isolation or alienation are diminished (Garnet and Douglas, 1993, 14). Research on gay men living with HIV has found that they have significantly better mental health than women and heterosexual men living with HIV. McDowell and Serovich (2007, 1227) argue that this is due to gay men developing and having access to larger social networks and communities where there are perceptions of sound support. Hunter et al. support these findings in their focus upon lesbian, gay and bisexual youths and adults. In coming out and developing a sense of identity, acceptance of sexual identity is linked to the ability to access positive support groups, resources and meet other men and women 'just like them'. These experiences allow lesbians, gay men and bisexuals to combat and challenge societal heterosexism and the potential mental health problems that heterosexism and homophobia can create (1998, 22–3).

Methodology

The data from which this chapter draws upon is from ESRC funded PhD research that was concerned with the experiences of lesbians and gay men of everyday city spaces in Newcastle.[6] A number of factors were felt to be of key importance in deciding who to recruit for the research sample. Three key factors, gender, age and social class were of central concern in ensuring diversity within the interviewees, with these having consequences for how the sample was accessed (see Casey, 2004; 2007). Identity development across the life course changes an individual's relationship with their peers, family and sexual identity (see Hunter et al., 1998; Varley and Blasco, 2001; Gorman-Murray, 2008). For example, younger lesbians and gay men are more likely to be living within the parental home or in shared accommodation. If they are not out about their sexual identity they may experience the home as oppressive that can create mental health concerns (see Ueno, 2005). Older lesbians and gay men are much more likely to have their own home spaces, although some may be married and others afraid of neighbours finding out about their sexual identity, which again can have profound impacts on mental health (Nordenmark and Stattin, 2009). Three age bands were created placing eight people in each (four men, four women, with a total of 23 participants).[7] The age groups were 18–25, 26–40 and 41+. These groups were chosen as they were felt to reflect three key life stages of 'youth', 'middle adulthood' and 'the older years'.[8] However, it is acknowledged that creating and placing individuals into such age specific groups and the giving these groups meaning can be problematic (see Weeks, 1981). As Nordenmark and Sattin (2009, 413) comment, age and experiences so associated are not a uniform process.

The socio-economic position of participants was also understood as an important factor in the development of the research sample. Socio-economic class has a significant impact upon the material wealth of individuals and in turn potential financial worries (or lack of) concerning finances (see Sorensen and Roberts, 1997; Liddle, 1999). In each of the three age groups of the eight members to be placed within each, four were chosen who self-identified as 'working class' and four who self-identified as 'middle class'. Understandings offered around class identity are complex and problematic (see Reay, 2001; Taylor, 2007), consequently,

---

6 Much research has previously centred upon large urban areas with significant lesbian and gay populations such as London (Binnie, 1995), Manchester (Quilley, 1997), New York (Dangerous Bedfellows, 1996), Los Angeles (Retter, 1997) or Sydney (Connell, 2000). Marc Lewis (1994) was the first to draw attention to 'gay Newcastle' positioning the city as being characteristically homophobic, rendering any lesbian or gay cultures as 'invisible' (see Casey, 2004; 2007).

7 Both the lesbian and gay male 18–25 age group had three lesbians and three gay men in each due to difficulties in getting this age group involved within the research. In the lesbian group of 26–40 there was five women placed within this due to a strong influence from lesbians in this age range to be involved.

8 Through the selecting of these age bands it was felt the groups would reflect the cultural and social changes within the UK such as British culture pre-1967 Sexual Offences Act, experiences of the gay liberation movement and lesbian feminism in the 1970s, the AIDS crisis in the 1980s and recent shifts which have affected lesbian and gay visibility and the place of sexual others in UK society.

understandings of 'working class' and 'middle class' in the research project were to be self-defined by respondents, with most respondents citing occupational background(s) as the reason for the claiming of a specific class position.

The research sample was accessed in five ways. Firstly bars on the lesbian and gay scene were targeted with flyers with information regarding the research. Following this, details of the research were published within the city based magazines '*The North Guide*' and '*The Crack*'. Next both lesbian and gay social/ support groups within Newcastle were approached, with feedback from the gay men's groups that were contacted being very good, although feedback from the lesbian support and social groups was poor.[9] The most significant source of interest came through working in Newcastle PRIDE. A number of those interested at PRIDE eventually developed as key contacts over the last few months of the interviews. The role of the key contacts was crucial in facilitating the recruitment of female respondents. Although my identity as a gay man surely facilitated my accessing of some of the respondents, my difficulty in recruiting respondents, in particular lesbians and older gay men, indicates the limits of sexual identity in acting as a common denominator (see Browne, Brown and Lim, 2007). For other respondents my assumed social class, age or gender may have been more important than my sexual identity alone.

In this research those in the sample lived within the city's suburbs of Jesmond and Heaton in the East of the city and Fenham in the West of the city. Jesmond can be characterised through its affluence, close proximity to the city centre and a mix of middle class residents and wealthy students. Heaton, although close to Jesmond is less affluent (and less expensive), attracting a mix of residents such as middle income young professionals, young families, students, local working class life-long residents of the area, and may be characterised by liberal attitudes and strong diversity. Fenham, the most ethnically diverse of the three neighbourhoods is characterised through a mix of low to mid income residents comprising students, young professionals and families.

Respondents were interviewed using qualitative semi-structured interviews. A number of key themes were used to structure the interviews, such as 'scene spaces', 'public space' and 'the home'. Each theme developed from existing literature upon the spatial experiences of lesbians and gay men and mental health concerns (e.g. Bell and Valentine, 1995; Hunter et al., 1998; Bruaner, 2000; Moran and Skeggs, 2004). It is hoped the quotes drawn upon below will allow professionals and practitioners to appreciate the diverse realities of lesbians and gay men, and the potential costs and benefits these quotidian realities have for lesbian's and gay men.

---

9   Lack of feedback from the lesbian social/support groups could possibly have been a consequence of myself (as the sole interviewer) identifying as a gay male, with the desire to provide anonymity and safety for members possibly being compromised.

Inclusions/Exclusions in the Lesbian and Gay Scene

The intersecting of ageism with gender, heterosexism and homophobia combines to construct a particularly negative stereotype of older lesbians and gay men (Hunter et al., 1998). In the latter part of the twentieth century and early twenty-first, the fear of becoming old within western societies has intensified significantly. Padva, (2002, 290) in reflecting upon the opinions of her gay male interviewees claims: 'they all blame the media, including the gay orientated media … for nurturing the muscular body and/or imagery of youth and youngness'. The domination of the youthful body as exclusively sexually desirable and attractive within popular cultural (Western) discourse has the consequence that those who can no longer at least *appear* to be 'youthful' are positioned as sexually undesirable. This focus on youthfulness, especially within the gay male scene (see Hunter et al., 1998; Casey, 2007) can create immense pressures on gay men to maintain their looks and bodies. The existence of older lesbians and gay men for Pugh (2002), have been largely sidetracked in the study of mental health and lesbian and gay sexuality. Much work (e.g. Casey, 2002; Ueno, 2005) is focused upon lesbian and gay youth, coming out stories or adult lesbians and gay men – rarely are retired or aged lesbians and gay men and their mental health needs addressed. Such a lack of work continues to underpin the assumption that a 'stable' sexual identity position will be achieved in later life or potential issues around sex, substance abuse, income or relationships are not the concerns of the elderly (see Weeks, 1981; Heaphy and Yip, 2006). Older lesbians and gay men for Pugh (2002) have been largely ignored by sexuality studies and social gerontology. However, such a focus on the young and their 'perfect and youthful' bodies also has consequences for those gay men and lesbians with disabilities. For a scene focused around drink, drugs, music and dancing (see Browne et al., 2007) for those with limited mobility, sight or hearing, full inclusion within scene spaces can be denied. As a reader myself of the gay press for the last 15 years I cannot re-call one image of a gay man who could be identified as having a disability. And as a number of the lesbians in this research discussed, deaf lesbians wishing to use sign language in Newcastle's only lesbian venue were unable to do so due to low light levels. Disability through its intersecting with sexuality reminds practitioners that people with disabilities are sexual, have sexual identities and face complex issues of inclusion/exclusion within gay, lesbian and heterosexual commercial sites where sexual partners are usually met (see Shakespeare, 1996; 2003). For those gay men and lesbians who are unable to claim an inclusion in scene spaces or the wider lesbian and gay community due to age, disability or due to limited incomes, the consequences for mental health can be severe.

In accessing and using lesbian and gay commercial sites, the ability to be openly out, meet friends and express affection to a partner, are cited as particular reasons for gaining access to such spaces (Knopp, 1995; Valentine, 2002; Brown, Lim and Browne, 2007). However since the mid 1990s many commercial scenes have been increasingly stylised, branded and marketed towards the youth market (see Skeggs,

1999, Moran and Skeggs, 2004), where identities other than sexual identity are affecting access to such sites. As I have discussed previously, (see Casey, 2007) movement into, from and the occupying of lesbian and gay commercial space(s) is increasingly restricted for those deemed to be the 'undesirable other'. The aged, disabled or poor looking body can mark out lesbians and gay men as 'undesirable others' whose movement into and use of such spaces has become increasingly restricted. Such emerging exclusions can have potential costs for feelings of inclusion and mental health concerns. As tolerance and acceptance of lesbian and gay men has increased in a number of western cultures the media has adopted the young, beautiful, white, wealthy and urban lesbian and/or gay man to represent the acceptable and desirable face of the sexual other. As one of Padva's (2002, 290) interviewees claimed 'gay magazines[:] it's all young and slim or big and muscular'. The gay male subculture in particular is youth orientated, although this is not an essentialist characteristic, but the result of intensive commercialisation, branding and value given to youthfulness and the 'body beautiful'. The aged body now has limited value within British culture, in turn mid-life and even more advanced years may present gay men with a crisis of confidence and identity, with anxiety developing about the loss of sexual attractiveness and/or sexual performance.[10] Views of older women in western cultures are generally more negative than they are for older men – this has consequences for older lesbians as women and as lesbians (Hunter et al., 1998: 156). For the older lesbian, lack of comfort in entering venues where younger lesbians and/or gay men are present may result in self-exclusion from certain sites as Liz and Margaret[11] reflect:

> I think there is a certain set, or certain group that is very body conscious and I suppose that puts quite a bit of pressure on you and that goes with the desire for eternal youth. (Liz, 30)

> I think the pubs and clubs in the city are *very* loud and *very* much aimed at young people … and it just occurred to me recently that I am probably too old for that anyway. (Margaret, 46)

Both Liz and Margaret reflect the intensification of 'youthfulness' on the scene, and the intense pressures this can create along with feelings of exclusion. As Margaret reflects 'I am probably too old for that anyway', with Liz echoing that

---

10   However, Pugh (2002, 164) suggests that the media presentation of Viagra has begun to challenge the assumption that a major user group of this drug – older men – do not have sex. Through the media's attention to Viagra older men's and consequently heterosexual women's desire for sex is increasingly entering everyday popular discourse. However the implication that older men need chemical enhancement to develop an erection and have sex has done little to challenge ideas of 'dirty old men' and the widespread belief within contemporary culture that only the young can/should have sex.

11   All names of interviewees and venues used within this chapter are pseudonyms.

the body consciousness and desire for 'eternal youth' of other clientele 'puts quite a bit of pressure on you'. Sorensen and Roberts (1997, 47) suggest that a focus on youthfulness is also a concern of heterosexual women, not one unique to lesbians or gay men alone. However the highly limited number of lesbian and gay venues in any city means older lesbians or gay men do not have easy access to alternative venues should one be 'too old' for its client base. Such pressure can create anxiety about physical appearance, 'fitting in' and meeting a potential partner, which Berg et al. (2008, 295) argue maybe be factors for the higher rates of mental health problems associated with gay men. For Chris, who is in his late fifties, in discussing his own experience of venues located within the Newcastle gay scene, his recent coming out and claims to a gay male identity position did not allow him experience feelings of inclusion and/or comfort in a number of gay identified venues:

> Well they [other clientele] were much younger than me, but most people are younger than me! And it became an issue after a while, as the longer you were there you thought this isn't my age, and this isn't my age group ... it is almost like saying I don't belong there. (Chris, 59)

Chris' discomfort and sense of 'I don't belong here', in the 'young venue' indicates that sexual identity is but one of a number of 'identities' or criteria that influence feelings of inclusion, belonging and/or comfort in a commercialised gay space. Participants in research by Ruth Holiday expressed unease and feelings of being evaluated, judged and/or not belonging when going out on the 'gay scene' (Holliday, 1999, 482). The experiences discussed here by Chris reflect how age and the aged body affect his ability to engage or connect with the venue he enters and the younger clientele. Although he has the financial ability to access the venue, his visible identity as an older gay man creates feelings of discomfort and unease for him. His suggestion that 'I don't belong there' echoes those claims often made by young lesbians and gay men as they experience coming out, finding a peer group and friendship networks. Research by those such as Hunter et al. (1998) and Berg et al. (2008) found that feelings of not belonging for older lesbians and gay men can have serious affects on mental health and suicidal tendencies. Research by those such as Saghir and Robins (1973) and Dawson (1982) found that although very few gay men actually grow old in isolation, many gay men report worrying about being 'alone' or not belonging in youth obsessed gay scenes. As Saghir and Robins (1973) found, only 28 per cent of their gay male respondents believed that they would have a partner in their older years. Kelly (1975) found that many gay men held negative beliefs about ageing, but as ageing began these beliefs declined. Of course, much of this work was undertaken in the 1970s, long before the intense proliferation of media images of youth and beauty.

This growing focus on 'youthfulness' was experienced as problematic for those no longer considered as being 'youthful' (or at least 'youthful' as defined by door staff, bar workers, venue owners, other clientele and/or as defined by themselves), creating previously unknown age restrictions, discomfort and exclusions for accessing venues in Newcastle's commercial gay district. This lack of access can then limit access to social networks. Research by Berger (1982) and Berger and Kelly (1996) found that older lesbians and gay men with high integration with gay scenes had lower incidences of poor mental health, were less fearful of ageing, more accepting and less depressed. Equally such lesbians and gay men were found to be more positive towards the worth and value of their sexual identity (see Quam and Whitford, 1992). However for some of the research sample, access and inclusion within the commercial scene was discussed as problematic:

> Because the others are SO loud! I just feel so old saying that! "Violins", you go there and you just feel like you are 140 years old! ...well "Violins" is alright, it's me that feels 140... (Kath, 40)

> ... pubs are kind of segregating people. "SIMS" has become the skinheads and the older crowd, I'm not too sure about upstairs, but downstairs it is very male orientated. 'The Cat', has become female orientated upstairs, "Thirst" has become the younger crowd, the drag queens and the older guys in "The House" and some of the students, it is kind of segregating slowly. (Matt, 22)

> ... it's very much geared towards younger people. A lot of my friends are older than me – you know, 35+. "The House" has made a big difference I have to say ... as "The House" is one place that you can actually hear yourself think. (Lauren, 23)

Work by Sarah Thornton in her study of British club and bar culture reminds us that door-staff have the power to inform potential club users if they are too old or too young, in turn denying access at the point of entry (Thornton, 1995). For those who do gain entry, feelings of comfort and/or inclusion can be fulfilled or denied through the type of music played, through to the ability to get served by younger bar staff. Matt's reflection upon the growing segregation between venues in larger urban areas may not be such a serious issue, where scenes are diverse and can cater for multiple niche markets. However, Newcastle, and other small cities and towns have a limit upon what they can offer their lesbian and gay residents, which may become increasingly limited as bar owners' chase the pink and very youthful pound. For Lauren, the lack of loud music in 'The House' and the presence of 'people their age' are understood to reflect that the venue is targeting 'older' lesbians and gay men. Although 'The House' may cater for those no longer considered 'youthful' on the lesbian and gay scene, her comment can also be understood as reflecting the growing commodification of gay spaces that removes spaces for political activism, support and/or comfort. The importance of youthfulness on the gay scene may be nothing new, in November 1977 the *Christopher Street* periodical was asking its readers '*where do all the old gays go?*', with a poster in mid-1980s Toronto echoing this question in asking '*what happens to homosexuals over 50?*' Pugh argues that the sentiments expressed here are as valid, if not more so, in the early twenty first century (2002, 162) as echoed by many of the research participants who discussed how the venues in the Newcastle scene were increasingly focused upon catering for a 'youth market' (see Jones and Pugh, 2005). Even if an upper age limit is not enforced by a venue, 'if you are not young and pretty', you can still feel excluded (Binnie, 1995, 198). However, work by Adelman (1991) may suggest that a decreased engagement with the gay scene is better for the mental health of older lesbians and gay men. His research reported that those who had less contact with other lesbians and gay men in their 'older years' had better mental health, although Hunter et al. (1998) suggest that most work contradicts these findings.

Home Spaces

In their discussion of 'home' Allan and Crow (1989) offer an understanding of home as a valued place in which members of a family can live in private, away from the scrutiny of others, and exercise control over outsider's involvement in domestic affairs' (1989, 4). As Young (2005) has also found, privacy, control, safety and support are all closely related in experiences and meanings of home. Such meanings and experiences are central to the home being a site of sanctuary from daily stressors and a place that can nurture and support sound mental well being (Berg et al., 2008). But, these approaches to home do not acknowledge the potential scrutiny, surveillance, harassment and intrusion within homes and of their occupants by 'outsiders', and the severe consequences this can have for mental well being. Equally, such an approach to home does not engage with the idea of potential control and violence from within the home from other residents. The work of Bornstein et al. (2006) and Murray and Mobley (2009) has shown the intersecting of violence, power and control within the lesbian, gay, bisexual and trans home – where domestic violence polices the identities and daily lives of its victims. Such work is moving discourses around domestic violence and the physical and mental consequences of it away from heterosexual relationships only. For lesbians and gay men and their home spaces, the ability of neighbours to read signifiers of their lesbian or gay male identity/ies (correctly or incorrectly) may have no negative consequences. However, should these be witnessed or read by the wrong neighbour in the wrong neighbourhood results can be severe. Homophobia can act as a push factor in the movement of lesbians and gay men to other locations perceived and characterised as more diverse or tolerant. Such homophobia can be seen as attempts to restore the respectability of the neighbourhood by driving the occupants out of the street (Harry, 1992). Research participants in studies by Lynch (1987) and Rothenberg (1995) reported that they gained prior knowledge through friends about areas of lesbian or gay tolerance before moving. Formal and informal networks act as encouragement in the movement of individuals to specific areas as Kath claimed:

> ... specific to the area that I have chosen, there is a lot of diversity, I think it's not out of the ordinary for lesbians and gay men to be your neighbours. (Kath, 40)

If homophobia is experienced some lesbians and gay men may re-locate, although such movements maintain the hegemony of heterosexuality within an area. It is also important to acknowledge that not all lesbians or gay men possess sufficient knowledge, resources or capital to be able to move away and relocate. For such lesbians and gay men heterosexism and/or homophobia are daily realities to be endured in their place of residence. Such experiences have been mirrored in the experiences of ethnic minorities and the affects of racial harassment on housing choice (Bowes and Sim, 2002; Somerville and Steele, 2002). Home can then become a place of isolation from the wider neighbourhood, with homophobia taking its toll on both mental and physical health. The ferocity of attacks and degree to which individuals are able to cope with them, can become central to surviving within homes that are targeted. Attacks upon a home can destroy feelings of comfort, ease and identity affirmation associated with feelings of 'being at home'. During the research this was indicated within a number of accounts. Both Eileen and Owen suffered homophobic attacks and abuse directed at them and their homes, although the degree of these varied:

> There are people who keep trashing my car and the police think it is because I am a lesbian. Well it's just a natural reaction now, I get up and make sure me car is alright and then I get ready and everything. Otherwise I have got to get me car sorted as I work freelance ... it usually happens around winter time, sort of every week, sometimes 2 or 3 times a week ... it's a window being put through here, somebody has shit on my windscreen. One time it happened 29 times within 31 days and every window day by day had been broken and every tyre had been slashed. And Christmas Eve they came and took me battery out me car. (Eileen, 41)

Living in a low-income neighbourhood of council housing, Eileen found her neighbours to be supportive of her sexual identity, but it is the threats and violence from 'gangs of youths' from surrounding streets that police her lesbian identity. Although Eileen had a limited income, and would have found it difficult financially to move, her continued residence in her street is through her own choice not to be 'scared away' by a minority of people. Lesbians and gay men are not necessarily passive victims of homophobia. During her interview Eileen suggested that her large friendship network and service in a number of lesbian and gay organisations 'kept her sane' when attacks occurred, echoing similar research findings (see Moran and Skeggs, 2004). The severe homophobia directed at Eileen marks her home place as an 'acceptable' target. In further discussions of these attacks, Eileen strongly believes her lack of conforming to a feminine appearance instigated the homophobic violence. As she shows, gender identity is read to indicate sexual identity, if Eileen was to appear more feminine, we could ask, would these attacks have been instigated? Similar harrowing experiences were found by Smaile's (1994) in her research on lesbian home spaces. Equally, Gorman-Murray acknowledges that 'houses occupied by adult gay men and lesbians ... come under heteronormative regulation from surrounding communities, with properties targeted for anti-gay harassment and violence' (2007, 198). The lesbian or gay home place, standing alone within a homophobic neighbourhood can almost be experienced as a prison, damaging to lesbian or gay mental health and wellbeing (see Johnston and Valentine, 1995). As homophobia infiltrates the lesbian or gay home space, an individual's ability to emotionally cope with its effects can become highly strained, as can the impact upon relationships for those partners who share the home.

> ... well I had just had enough [of being gay] and AIDS and everything, this was the 1980s ... Anyway I met this girl through an organization and we were just friends, and we became closer. Then somebody got knowledge of me being gay and there was an investigation saying I was abusing her children and it was all ill founded ... And the police and stuff were involved ... but there was no case to answer. So as a result of that, there was issues, some teenage boys you know were calling us pervert, poof, you know? ... But at the time I thought about moving house, I almost had a nervous breakdown, 'cos I hadn't done anything wrong. It wasn't very nice you know? (Robert, 56)

Homophobic violence and abuse serve as violent reminders to other lesbians and gay men within the neighbourhood of the need to pass or hide their sexual identity if they are to avoid being the next target. For Robert the fluidity of his sexual identity, reflected in his move from gay male relationships to developing and maintaining a relationship with a woman and taking a parental role with her children, may have challenged taken for granted assumptions concerning 'fixed' sexual identities and what constitutes 'family' (see Hunt, 1989; Firat and Dholakia, 1998; Richardson, 2000). As with Eileen, Robert's neighbours are supportive of his relationship and his new parental role, where it is the casual 'passer by' who disrupts his home life and challenges his sexual identity. The severe consequences of this harassment for his mental health are reflected upon, in his near arrival at a nervous breakdown and the eventual collapse of his relationship. Due to Robert's weak financial situation he was to end up living in a hostel for homeless people, itself creating new concerns around other tenant's views on his sexual identity and the potential risks this creates.

Conclusion

The data drawn upon in this paper reflects the diverse realities of lesbians and gay men, where far from being a homogeneous group, their daily realities and in turn, mental health needs, are often unique. Literature upon and mental health practice with lesbians and gay men has improved significantly since the first edition of the *Diagnostic and Statistical Manual of Mental Disorders* (1952). Such a shift in approaches can be contributed to better understandings of sexual identities beyond heterosexuality and the rejection of the medicalised model of homosexuality – with lesbians and gay men naming and claiming of their own sexual identities. As the literature and data drawn upon in this chapter indicates, the unique mental health needs of lesbians and gay men must be attributed to wider societal homophobia, but also pressures from within the lesbian and gay communities themselves. The growing obsession by the lesbian and gay commercial scene and media around youthfulness has serious consequences for the ability of older lesbians and gay men to claim an inclusion and visibility within commercial sites. As other literature has shown (e.g. Dawson, 1982; Berg et al., 2008) along with the data presented here, this obsession with all things young has consequences for the mental health concerns of older lesbians and gay men. If lesbians and gay men are denied an inclusion within the spaces they once helped create, the consequences for their mental health as they age can be severe (Hunter et al., 1998). Equally the lesbian or gay home, a site of potential identity development and affirmation, can also contribute to serious mental health concerns when homophobic violence is used against the lesbian or gay resident. The ability of residents to cope will often be influenced by access to wider social networks, support off neighbours or the financial ability to move home to find a more secure and lesbian or gay friendly neighbourhood. The approach of mental health organisations and those professionals working within the discipline towards lesbians and gay men, has improved significantly. However such organisations and workers need to be aware of unique stressors that lesbians and gay men can experience and the potential impact of this for their mental health needs. A lesbian or gay sexual identity does not stand alone, but is influenced by and intersects with multiple identities in multiple spatial sites during the everyday lives of lesbians and gay men that have very real material consequences.

Bibliography

Abelson, J., Lambevski, S., Crawford, J., Bartos, M. and Kippax, S. (2006) 'Factors associated with "feeling suicidal": The role of sexual identity', *Journal of Homosexuality*. Vol. 51(1), pp. 59–80.

Adam, B.D. (2000) 'Love and sex in constructing identity among men who have sex with men', *International Journal of Sexuality and Gender Studies*. Vol. 5(4), pp. 325–339.

Adelman, M. (1991) 'Stigma, gay lifestyles and adjustment to ageing: A study of later-life gay men and lesbians', in Lee, J.A. (ed.), *Gay Midlife and Maturity*, pp. 1–32 (New York: Haworth Press).

Allan, G. and Crow, G. (1989) *Home and Family: Creating the Domestic Sphere* (London: Macmillan).

Altman, D. (2002) 'Globalization and the international gay/lesbian movement', Richardson, D. and Seidman, S. (eds), *Handbook of Lesbian and Gay Studies*, pp. 415–426. (London: Sage).

Avery, A.M., Hellman, R.R. and Sudderth, L.K. (2001) 'Satisfaction with mental health services among sexual minorities with major mental health illness', in *American Journal of Public Health*. Vol. 91(6), pp. 990–991.

Bailey, J.M. (1999) 'Homosexuality and mental illness', *Arch Gen Psychiatry*. Vol. 56(Oct), pp. 883–884.

Bawrer, B. (1994) *A Place at the Table* (New York: Touchstone).

Beasley, C. (ed.) (2005) *Gender and Sexuality: Critical Theories, Critical Thinkers* (London: Sage).

Bell, D. and Valentine, G. (eds) (1995) *Mapping Desire; Geographies of Sexualities* (London: Routledge).

Berg, M.B., Mimiaga, M.J. and Safren, S.A. (2008) 'Mental health concerns of Gay and bisexual men seeking mental health services', *Journal of Homosexuality*. Vol. 54(3), pp. 293–306.

Berger, R.M. (1982) 'The unseen minority: Older gays and lesbians', *Social Work*. 27, 236–242.

Berger, R.M. and Kelly, J.J. (1996) 'Gay men and lesbians grown old', in Cabaj, R.P. and Stein, T.S. (eds), *Textbook of Homosexuality and Mental Health*, pp. 305–316 (Washington, DC: American Psychiatric Press).

Binnie, J. (1995) 'Trading places: Consumption, sexuality and production of queer space', in Bell, D. and Valentine, G. (eds), *Mapping Desire: Geographies of Sexualities*, pp. 182–199 (London: Routledge).

Birke, L. (2002) 'Scientific studies of sexual orientation', in Richardson, D. and Seidman, S. (eds), *Handbook of Lesbian and Gay Studies*, pp. 55–72 (London: Sage).

Bowes, A. and Sim, D. (2002) 'Patterns of residential settlement among black and minority ethnic groups', in Summerville, P. and Steele, A. (eds), *Race, Housing and Social Exclusion*, pp. 40–60 (London: Jessica Kingsley Publisher).

Bristow, J. (ed.) (1993) *Activating Theory: Lesbian, Gay, Bisexual Politics* (London: Lawrence and Wishart).

Brookey, R.A. (2000) 'Saints or sinners: Sociobiological theories of male homosexuality', *International Journal of Sexuality and Gender Studies*. Vol. 5(1), pp. 37–58.

Brown, K., Lim, J. and Browne, G. (eds) (2007) *Geographies of Sexualities: Theory, Practice and Politics* (Aldershot: Ashgate).

Campos, P.E. and Goldfried, M.R. (2001) 'Introduction: Perspectives on therapy with gay, lesbian and bisexual clients', *Psychotherapy in Practice*. Vol. 57(5), pp. 609–613.

Casey, M. (2002) 'Young gay males experiences of coming out in the context of school', *Youth and Policy.* Spring, 75, pp. 62–75.

Casey, M. (2004) 'De-dyking queer spaces: Heterosexual female visibility in gay and lesbian spaces', *Sexualities*. Vol. 7(4), pp. 446–461.

Casey, M. (2007) 'The queer unwanted and their undesirable otherness', Brown, K., Lim, J. and Browne, G. (eds), *Geographies of Sexualities: Theory, Practice and Politics*, pp. 125–136 (Aldershot: Ashgate).

Casey, M. (2009) 'Addressing key theoretical approaches to gay male sexual identity: Issues and insights for practitioners of mental health', *Critical Public Health*. Vol. 19(3), pp. 12–24.

Cruishank. M. (1992) *The Gay and Lesbian Liberation Movement* (New York: Routledge & Kegan Paul).

Darius, S. and Johnson, S. (1993) 'Interview with Gayatri Spivak', *Boundary 2*. Vol. 20(2).

Davies, D. (1996) 'Towards a model of gay affirmative therapy', in Davies, D. and Neal, C. (eds), *Pink Therapy: A Guide for Counsellors and Therapists Working with Lesbians, Gay Men and Bisexual Clients* (Buckingham: Open University Press).

Davies, D. and Neal. C. (eds) (1996) *Pink Therapy: A Guide for Counsellors and Therapists Working with Lesbians, Gay Men and Bisexual Clients* (Buckingham: Open University Press).

Davies, D. and Neal, C. (eds) (2000) *Therapeutic Perspectives on Working with Lesbian, Gay and Bisexual Clients* (Buckingham: Open University Press).

Davison, G.C. (2001) 'Conceptual and ethical issues in therapy for the psychological problems of gay men, lesbians and bisexuals', *Psychotherapy in Practice*. Vol. 57(5), pp. 695–704.

Dawson, K. (1982) *Serving the Older Gay Community*, SIECUS Report November, 17, 5–6.

Diaz, R.M., Ayala, G., Bein, E., Henne, J. and Marin, B.V. (2001) 'The impact of homophobia, poverty and racism on the mental health of gay and bisexual latino men: Findings from 3 US cities', *American Journal of Public Health*. Vol. 91(6), pp. 927–932.

Engel, S. (2002) 'Making a minority: Understanding the formation of the gay and lesbian movement in the United States', in Richardson, D. and Seidman, S. (eds), *Handbook of Lesbian and Gay Studies*, pp. 375–402 (London: Sage).

Epstein, S. (1992) 'Gay politics, ethnic identity', in Stein, E. (ed.), *Forms of Desire* (New York: Routledge).

Fergusson, D.M., Horwood, J.L. and Beautrais, A.L. (1999) 'Is sexual orientation related to mental health problems and suicidality in young people?' *Arch Gen Psychiatry*. Vol. 56(Oct), pp. 876–880.

Foucault, M. (1978) *The History of Sexuality: Volume 1* (London: Penguin Books).

Foucault, M. (1992) 'The perverse implantation', in Stein, E. (ed.), *Forms of Desire: Sexual Orientation and the Social Constructionist Controversy*, pp. 11–23 (London: Routledge).

Gagnon, J. and Simon, W. (1973) *Sexual Conduct: The Social Sources of Human Sexuality* (London: Hutchinson).

Garnets, L.D. and Kimmel, D.C. (eds) (1993) *Psychological Perspectives on Lesbian and Gay Male Experiences* (New York: Columbia University Press).

Glazer, D.F., Guss, J.R., D'Ercole, A. and Masters, S. (2008) 'Homosexuality and psychoanalysis III: Clinical perspectives', *Journal of Gay and Lesbian Mental Health*. Vol. 12(4), pp. 355–379.

Gorman-Murray, A. (2007) Contesting domestic ideals: Queering the Australian home, *Australian Geographer*. Vol. 38(2), pp. 195–213.

Gorman-Murray, A. (2008) 'Reconciling self: Gay men and lesbians using domestic materiality for identity management', *Social and Cultural Geography*. Vol. 9(3), pp. 283–301.

Gray, J. (2000) 'Cognitive-behavioural therapy', in Davies, D. and Neal, C. (eds), *Therapeutic Perspectives on Working with Lesbian, Gay and Bisexual Clients*, pp. 24–38 (Buckingham: Open University Press).

Guardian, The (2008) 'Little pink book', *Guardian Travel*, p. 5 (28.06.08).

Halpert, S.C. (2000) 'If it ain't broke, don't fix it: Ethical considerations regarding conversion therapies', *International Journal of Sexuality and Gender Studies*. Vol. 5(1), pp. 19–35.

Hamer, D.H. (1993) 'The linkage between DNA markers on the x-chromosome and male sexual orientation', *Science*. Vol. 16:26(5119), pp. 321–327.

Harry, J. (1992) 'Conceptualising anti-gay violence', in Herek, G.M. and Berril, K.T. (eds), *Hate Crimes: Confronting Violence Against Lesbians and Gay Men* (London: Sage).

Hawkes, G. (1996) *Sociology and Social Change: The Sociology of Sex and Sexuality* (Buckingham: Open University Press).

Heaphy, B., Weeks, J. and Donovan, C. (eds) (1998) 'That's my life', *Sexualities*. Vol. 1(4), pp. 453–470.

Heaphy, B. and Yip, A.K.T (2006) 'Policy implications of ageing sexualities', *Social Policy and Society*. Vol. 5(4), pp. 443–451.

Herrel, R., Goldberg, J., True, W.R., Ramakrishnan, V., Lyons, M., Eisen, S. and Tsuang, M.T. (1999) 'Sexual orientation and suicidality', *Arch Gen Psychiatry*. Vol. 56(Oct), pp. 867–874.

Holliday, R. (1999) 'The comfort of identity', *Sexualities*. Vol. 2(4), pp. 475–491.

Hunter, S., Shannon, C., Knox, J. and Martin, J. (1998) *Lesbian, Gay and Bisexual Adults: Knowledge for Human Service Practice* (London: Sage).

Ingraham, C. (2002) 'Heterosexuality: It's just not normal!', in Richardson, D. and Seidman, S. (eds), *Handbook of Lesbian and Gay Studies*, pp. 73–81 (London: Sage).

Isay, R.A. (1989) *Being Homosexual: Gay Men and their Development* (New York: Avon Books).

Jackson, S. (1999) *Heterosexuality in Question* (London: Sage).

Jackson, S. and Weeks, J. (2005) 'Social constructionism', in Beasley, C. (ed.), *Gender and Sexuality: Critical Theories, Critical Thinkers*, pp. 135–143 (London: Sage).

Jones, J. and Pugh, S. (2005) 'Lessons from the sociology of embodiment', *Men and Masculinities*. Vol. 7(3), pp. 248–260.

Johnston, L. and Valentine, G. (1995) 'Wherever I lay my girlfriend that's my home: The performance and surveillance of lesbian identities in domestic environments', in Bell, D. and Valentine, G. (eds), *Mapping Desire: Geographies of Sexualities*, pp. 99–113 (London: Routledge).

Kaufman, J.S., Carlozzi, A.F., Boswell, D.L., Barnes, L., Wheeler-Scruggs, K. and Levy, P.A. (1997) 'Factors influencing therapist selection among gays, lesbians and bisexuals', *Counselling Psychology Quarterly*. Vol. 10(3), pp. 287–297.

Kelly, J. (1975) 'Brothers and brothers: The gay men's adaption of ageing' (Doctoral Dissertation, Brandeis University, 1974). *Dissertation Abstracts International*, 36, 3103A.

Koh, A. and Ross, L. (2006) 'Mental health issues: A comparison of lesbian, bisexual and heterosexual women', *Journal of Homosexuality*. Vol. 51(1), pp. 33–57.

Kort, J. (2008) *Gay Affirmative Therapy for the Straight Clinician – The Essential Guide* (New York: Norton).

Knopp, L. (1995) 'Sexuality and urban space: A framework for analysis', in Bell, D. and Valentine, G. (eds), *Mapping Desire: Geographies of Sexualities*, pp. 149–163 (London: Routledge).

LA Times (2008) 'What does gay look like? Science keeps trying to figure it out' <www.latimes.com> 16.06.08.

Le Vay, S. (1993) *The Sexual Brain* (Cambridge, MA: MIT Press).

Liddle, B.J. (1999) 'Recent improvement in mental health services to lesbian and gay clients', *Journal of Homosexuality*. Vol. 37(4), pp. 127–137.

Lynch, F.R. (1987) 'Non-ghetto gays: A sociological study of suburban homosexuals', *Journal of Homosexuality*. Vol. 13(4), pp. 13–42.

Maylon, A. (1982) 'Psychotherapeutic implications of internalized homophobia in gay men', in Gonsiorek, J. (ed.), *Homosexuality and Psychotherapy* (New York: Haworth Press).

McDowell, T.L. and Serovich, J.M. (2007) 'The effect of perceived and actual social support on mental health of HIV-positive persons', *AIDS Care*. Vol. 19(10), pp. 1223–1229.

McIntosh, M. (1968) 'The homosexual role', Reprinted in Nardi, P.M. and Schneider, B.E. (eds) (1998) *Social Perspectives in Lesbian and Gay Studies*, pp. 68–76 (London: Routledge).

Miller, M.L. (2008) 'Straight, gay, or both: The case of Michael', *Journal of Gay and Lesbian Mental Health*. Vol. 12(4), pp. 381–397.

Moon, L. (ed.) (2007) *Feeling Queer or Queer Feelings: Radical Approaches to Counselling Sex, Sexualities and Genders* (London: Routledge).

Moran, L. and Skeggs, B. (2004) *Sexuality and the Politics of Violence and Safety* (London: Routledge).

Nardi, P. (1992) 'That's what friends are for: Friends as family in the gay and lesbian community', in Plummer, K. (ed.), *Modern Homosexualities: Fragments of Lesbian and Gay Experience*, pp. 108–120 (London: Routledge).

Neal, C. and Davis, D. (eds) (2000) *Issues in Therapy with Lesbian, Gay, Bisexual and Transgender Clients* (Buckingham: Open University Press).

Nordenmark, M. and Stattin, M. (2009) 'Psychosocial wellbeing and reasons for retirement in Sweden', *Ageing and Society*. Vol. 29, pp. 413–430.

Nye, R.A. (1999) *Sexuality* (Oxford: Oxford University Press).

Ovesey, L. (1969) *Homosexuality and Pseudohomosexuality* (Northvale, New Jersey: Jason Aranson).

Padva, G. (2002) 'Heavenly monsters: The politics of the male body in the naked issue of *Attitude* Magazine', *International Journal of Sexuality and Gender Studies*. Vol. 7(4), pp. 281–292.

Pett, J. (2000) 'Gay, lesbian and bisexual therapy and its supervision', in Davies, D. and Neal, C. (eds), *Therapeutic Perspectives on Working with Lesbian, Gay and Bisexual Clients*, pp. 54–72 (Buckingham: Open University Press).

Plummer, K. (1981) *The Making of the Modern Homosexual* (New Jersey: Barnes and Noble Books).

Plummer, K. (ed.) (1992) *Modern Homosexualities: Fragments of Lesbian and Gay Experience* (London: Routledge).

Pugh, S. (2002) 'The forgotten: A community without a generation – older lesbians and gay men', in Richardson, D. and Seidman, S. (eds), *Handbook of Lesbian and Gay Studies* (London: Sage).

Quam. J.K. and Whitford, G.S. (1992) 'Adaption and age related expectations of older gay and lesbian adults', *Gerontologist*. Vol. 32, pp. 367–374.

Quzi, R. (2008) *Scans see 'Gay Brain Differences'* <bbcnews.co.uk> 17.06.08.

Rado, S. (1969) *Adaptational Psychodynamics: Motivation and Control* (New York: Science House).

Reay, D. (2001) 'The double-bind of the "working class" feminist academic: The success of failure or the failure of success?', in Arrighi, B.A. (ed.), *Understanding Inequality: The Intersection of Race/Ethnicity, Class and Gender*, pp. 76–82 (Oxford: Rowman and Littlefield Publishers Inc.).

Richardson, D. (1987) 'Recent challenges to traditional assumptions about homosexuality: Some implications for practice', in *Journal of Homosexuality*. Vol. 13(4), pp. 1–41.

Richardson, D. (2000) *Rethinking Sexuality* (London: Sage).

Richardson, D. (2004) 'Locating sexualities: From here to normality', *Sexualities*. Vol. 7(4), pp. 391–411.

Richardson, D. and Seidman, S. (eds) (2002) *Handbook of Lesbian and Gay Studies* (London: Sage).

Richardson, D., McLaughlin, J. and Casey, M.E. (eds) (2006) *Intersections Between Feminist and Queer Theory* (Basingstoke: Palgrave Macmillan).

Rothenberg, T. (1995) 'And she told two friends: Lesbians creating urban social space', in Bell, D. and Valentine, G. (eds), *Mapping Desire: Geographies of Sexualities*, pp. 165–181 (London: Routledge).

Safren, S.A. and Rogers, T. (2001) 'Cognitive-behavioural therapy with gay, lesbian and bisexual clients', *Psychotherapy in Practice*. Vol. 57(5), pp. 629–643.

Saghir, M.T. and Robins, E. (1973) *Male and Female Homosexuality* (Baltimore: Williams and Williams).

Sandfort, T.G.M., de Graaf, R., Bijl, R.V. and Schnabel, P. (2001) 'Same-sex sexual behaviour and psychiatric disorders: Findings from the Netherlands Mental Health Survey and Incidence Study', *Arch Gen Psychiatry*. Vol. 58(Jan), pp. 85–91.

Sandfort, T.G.M., Bakker, F., Schellevis, F.G. and Vanwesenbeeck, I. (2006) 'Sexual orientation and mental and physical health status: Findings from a Dutch population study', *American Journal of Public Health*. Vol. 96(6), pp. 1119–1125.

Segal, L. (1997) 'Sexualities', in Woodward, K. (ed.), *Identity and Difference*, pp. 184–238 (London: Open University Press and Sage).

Seidman, S., Fischer, N. and Meeks, C. (eds) (2007) *Introducing the New Sexuality Studies* (London: Routledge).

Shakespeare, T. (1996) 'Power and prejudices: Issues of gender, sexuality and disability', in Barton, L. (ed.), *Disability and Society: Emerging Issues and Insights*, pp. 191–214 (London: Longman).

Shakespeare, T. (2003) '"I haven't seen that in the Kama Sutra": The sexual stories of disabled people', in Weeks, J., Hollands, J. and Waites, M. (eds), *Sexuality and Society: A Reader*, pp. 143–152 (Cambridge: Polity Press).

Simon, G. and Whitfield, G. (2000) 'Social constructionist and systemic therapy', in Davies, D. and Neal, C. (eds), *Therapeutic Perspectives on Working with Lesbian, Gay and Bisexual Clients*, pp. 144–162 (Buckingham: Open University Press).

Skeggs, B. (1999) 'Matter out of place: Visibility and sexualities in leisure spaces', *Leisure Studies*. Vol. 18(3), pp. 213–222.

Smailes, J. (1994) 'The struggle has never been simply about bricks and mortar: Lesbian's experiences of housing', in Gilroy, R. and Woods, R. (eds), *Housing Women*, pp. 152–172 (London: Routledge).

Sorenson, L. and Roberts, S.J. (1997) 'Lesbian uses of and satisfaction with mental health services: Results from Boston Lesbian Health Project', *Journal of Homosexuality*. Vol. 33(1), pp. 35–49.

Stein, E. (ed.) (1992) *Forms of Desire: Sexual Orientation and the Social Constructionist Controversy* (London: Routledge).

Summerville, P. and Steele, A. (eds) (2002) *Race, Housing and Social Exclusion* (London: Jessica Kingsley Publishers).

Taylor, Y. (2007) *Working Class Lesbian Life: Classed Outsiders* (London: Palgrave Macmillan).

Thornton, S. (1995) *Club Cultures: Music, Media and the Subcultural Capital* (Cambridge: Polity Press).

Ueno, K. (2005) 'Sexual orientation and psychological distress in adolescence: Examining interpersonal stressors and social support processes', *Social Psychology Quarterly*. Vol. 68(3), pp. 258–277.

Valentine, G. (2002) 'Queer bodies and the production of space', in Richardson, D. and Seidman, S. (eds), *Handbook of Lesbian and Gay Studies*, pp. 145–160 (London: Sage).

Vance, C. (1992) 'Social construction theory: Problems in the history of sexuality', in Crowley, H. and Himmelweit, S. (eds), *Knowing Women: Feminism and Knowledge* (Oxford: Polity Press).

Varley, A.R. and Blasco, M. (2001) 'Exiled to the home: Masculinity and ageing in urban Mexico', *European Journal of Development Research*. Vol. 12(4), pp. 115–138.

Waters, A.T. (1986) 'Heterosexual bias in psychological research on lesbianism and male homosexuality (1979–1983), utilizing the bibliographic and taxonomic system of Morin (1977)', *Journal of Homosexuality*. Vol. 13(1), pp. 35–58.

Weeks, J. (1981) 'The problem of older homosexuals', in Hart, J. and Richardson, D. (eds), *The Theory and Practice of Homosexuality*, pp. 177–184 (London: Routledge & Kegan Paul).

Weeks, J. (1989) *Sex, Politics and Society: The Regulation of Sexuality Since 1800* (London: Longman).

Weeks, J. (2000) *Making Sexual History* (Oxford: Polity Press).

Weeks, J., Holland, J. and Waites, M. (2003) *Sexuality and Society: A Reader* (Oxford: Polity Press).

Williams, W.L. (1987) 'Women, men and others: Beyond ethnocentrism in gender theory', *American Behavioural Scientist*. Vol. 31, pp. 135–141.

Young, I.M. (2005) 'House and home: Feminist variations on a theme', in Young, I.M. (ed.), *On Female Body Experience: Throwing Like a Girl and Other Essays*, pp. 123–154 (New York: Oxford University Press).

Chapter 9

Beyond Cisgenderism: Counselling People with Non-Assigned Gender Identities

Y. Gavriel Ansara

Introduction: Why Equal Treatment Isn't Enough

As the Founding Director of Lifelines Rhode Island/Cuerdas de Salvamento, a regional non-profit organisation focused on meeting the needs of individuals with *non-assigned gender identities*,[1] I provided advocacy, support, referrals, and crisis intervention services to hundreds of individuals with extremely diverse demographic characteristics and needs. My position also involved conducting professional training programmes and offering consulting services for physicians, psychologists, educators, clergy, and other human service providers. This position gave me intimate views into the daily lives of many individuals and the myriad elements affecting their lives. During this time, my other day job involved working in the editorial office of an internationally recognised, peer-reviewed psychology journal. The stark contrast between the understandings I gained during my work at Lifelines and the inaccurate, disparaging depictions of our constituents[2] in psychological literature that I encountered at the journal revealed a wide gap between clinician awareness and service user experiences.

During an interactive component of a Continuing Education training exercise that I was conducting with a group of mental health professionals, one woman was brave enough to raise a question that echoed concerns others later said they had felt uncomfortable asking aloud: 'I treat all of my clients equally and like human beings. Why do I have to know how to treat trans and gender variant clients? I just treat everyone the same; I respect and understand them. Why do I need this training?'

---

1 People whose gender identities differ from those they were assigned; often termed people with affirmed genders or people of trans, intersex, and/or non-binary gender experience, e.g., a person with an *assigned* gender identity as a man who identifies as a woman can be described as a *woman with a non-assigned gender identity or* an *affirmed woman.*

2 During my tenure, Lifelines used the term 'constituents' to emphasise that persons served were stakeholders whose lived experiences and feedback motivated frequent revisions of our policies, procedures, and informational materials. *Constituent* implies civic engagement rather than consumerism.

I discovered that the 'Why is this necessary, anyway?' sentiment was widespread among participants in my trainings. This also included staff at nominally gay, lesbian, and bisexual agencies, who felt that the mere addition of a 'T' to their identifying acronym in the form of 'LGBT' prepared them sufficiently for responding to individuals with trans-related concerns.[3] I also encountered counsellors of trans experience who felt that their personal experiences enabled them to utter authoritative pronouncements to their colleagues about ideal professional responses to All Trans People Everywhere.

Numerous texts aspire to be complete reference guides on this topic or offer monolithic guidelines for counselling trans and non-binary gender clients. Yet psychological texts and training manuals rarely consider the tremendous variety of situational permutations that affect the daily lives of individuals with non-assigned gender identities. I say 'individuals' because neither my personal experience of gender affirmation nor my extensive involvement in trans-only social networks prepared me sufficiently for the dazzling array of perspectives and experiences that I encountered during my tenure as Lifelines director.

This chapter addresses the question 'Why is this necessary?' in a manner that I hope will initiate meaningful critical dialogue and reflexivity for counsellors regarding their clinical judgements and service delivery, a point of departure for future insights. The tendency of many authors in this field to impose academic and theoretical viewpoints that ignore or negate the complexities and incongruities of actual people's lives is one reason I have chosen to focus on the individuals whose lives touched mine when making conceptual points in this chapter.

In this chapter, I will use the term cisgenderism[4] to describe the individual, social, and institutional attitudes, policies, and practices that assume people with non-assigned gender identities are inferior, 'unnatural' or disordered and which construct people with non-assigned gender identities as 'the effect to be explained'.[5] This definition of cisgenderism offers a new paradigm for understanding currents that run through the vignettes that follow. My theoretical framework has been placed in the concluding section rather than at the beginning of this chapter because I believe that meaningful theory must emerge from the front lines of the people it claims to represent rather than from within clinical or ivory tower academic disciplinary boundaries.

---

3   The terms 'gay', 'lesbian', and 'bisexual' describe sexual orientation, not gender identity. Sexual orientation, sometimes termed affectional orientation, refers to people's erotic attractions, romantic partner preferences, and/or kinship ties.

4   Originally from *cisgender* (Buijs, 1996), but see Serano, 2007 for an examination of *cisgenderism*. The prefix *cis-* is derived from Latin, meaning "on the same side". For example, in organic chemistry, the phrase *cis-trans* isomerism is used to designate contrasting structural formulas in compounds with identical molecular formulae.

5   See Hegarty and Pratto, 2001 for an explanation of norms and 'the effect to be explained'.

I have selected merely a small sample of situations out of the hundreds of situations that I encountered. Rather than issue blanket pronouncements or propose a single method for streamlining counselling responses to people of trans experience, I have chosen to illustrate absurdities and inadequacies of current policies and practice – indeed, of any attempt to impose a normative policy or practice in this field – and to share an array of techniques that my volunteers and I found effective and beneficial. This chapter is my attempt to answer the aforementioned 'Why is this necessary?' question in a manner that will initiate meaningful critical dialogue for counsellors regarding their clinical judgements and service delivery. Numerous relevant topics have been omitted or only minimally addressed by this chapter and by available literature. Yet my intention is to provide a point of departure rather than the detrimental illusion of fluency that predominates in our field.

Beyond What Meets the Eye

I first encountered Danielle[6] on the telephone. She was afraid to meet in person. After several phone calls, her voice trembled as she agreed to meet with me and one of my Peer Advocates in the office space Lifelines had just acquired in the back room of a local print shop. Extremely concerned about her privacy, she insisted upon changing out of her flannel lumberjack shirt in the tiny bathroom beside the back entrance before meeting with us. She emerged wearing a modest peach pantsuit and low heels, her pink lipstick matching the smile that hovered uncertainly at the corners of her mouth. Her gaze flitted briefly from the floor to our staff and then back down, her hands shaking as she smoothed her hands across the hem of her blouse. The peer advocate and I smiled encouragingly, honoured to bear witness to her as she presented herself as she wished to be seen by others for the first time in over 50 years. Unfortunately, the owner of the print shop picked that moment to allow a 12-year-old boy into the back room. The multiple conversations with me and my clinical supervisor about the extreme privacy needs of our constituents and the importance of not allowing his customers into our space while we were in meetings had failed. The boy glared at Danielle for several long moments, while her hands shook with increasing rapidity, her smile faltering as I began collecting Lifelines' newly placed office supplies for removal in front of her to reassure her that we would not retain office space in a hostile environment, a tangible assurance that her safety was more important to us than this particular office space. My willingness to relinquish an asset as vital as office space when retaining that asset became incompatible with Danielle's best interests highlights the secondary marginalisation and sacrifices that counsellors may face while trying to maintain ethical practices.

---

6 Names and identifying details of all individuals mentioned in this chapter have been altered to the extent necessary to protect their privacy.

As Danielle invited us into her life, she taught me that, despite my own experience of having a non-assigned gender identity and the fact that local professionals were beginning to consider me an expert in All Things Trans, all of us had a lot to learn. One of the first insights most people gain when working with people who are exploring non-assigned gender identities is the importance of pronouns; 'she' or 'he', 'him or her'. Typically, ideas about appropriate pronoun usage are limited to identifying a person who appears visually ambiguous to the viewer and either assiduously avoiding gendered pronoun usage or asking which pronoun the person prefers. The former is frequently experienced as degrading or insulting by individuals with a clear pronoun preference, while the latter can often attract the unwanted attention of others who are present, and both cases can result in a sense of social exclusion. Nonetheless, assigning a pronoun based on social categorisation of visual appearance is risky – risky in the sense that an incorrect assignment can damage client trust. Constituents like Danielle provided me with the insight to see that the usage of pronouns and gendered terminology was even more complex than I had anticipated. This complexity also extends to matters of attire and visual presentation.

The single parent of a young child, Danielle struggled with the competing demands of caring for her terminally ill spouse, finding safe ways to simultaneously express her gender identity and maintain her family. Since her wardrobe of women's clothes had been discovered, Danielle's strict Christian relatives had threatened to seek full custody of her child if she demonstrated any signs of continuing to express her gender as a woman, an expression that they considered psychologically abnormal, dangerous, and deviant.

After hearing about her extreme isolation, I invited her to attend the support group that I facilitated for people articulating, exploring, or affirming non-assigned gender identities. She stressed that if we encountered her outside of the group, we must address her as Jack and use male pronouns. This was not due to gender ambiguity or hesitation on her part; she was petrified that someone from her insular, rural community might discover her identity and try to destroy her family. It was a learning experience for the members of the group to witness Danielle attending the group with the thick, coarse arm hair, stubble, and flannel shirts typically associated with men, looking every bit the part of the robust lumberjack she had to be to sustain her home life, while being referred to consistently as Danielle and 'she'. Danielle's presence reminded all of us that the freedom to present as a member of the gender with which one identifies – *despite* one's attire, hair, voice, or mannerisms – was a basic human right denied to many others in similarly repressive situations. For other group members, fear of governmental and police oppression deterred them from exercising this right; despite the inclusion of trans individuals in local equal protection legislation, these laws were rarely known or observed by local police, who routinely harassed and arrested numerous women from our group for illegal sex work solely because they did not 'pass'[7] as female when wearing women's clothes in public.

For Danielle, the group was a respite from the oppressive act she was compelled to play in daily life, the stress of a role that did not match her inner longings. Sometimes, I would arrive early enough to unlock the door in time for her to change into comfortable women's clothing prior to the meeting. At other times, she was barely able to abscond from the responsibilities of home and family for long enough to slip inside the building before our meetings were over. Yet each time she joined us, Danielle expressed relief that she had one safe place in which to explore what it felt like to be herself. Consequently, group sessions take on a critical role – they are perhaps the only setting in which some people experience the liberation of being 'seen' and 'heard', essential components of trauma recovery and transcending marginalisation. During the check-in period at the beginning of each meeting, after the ground rules were recited aloud by the group, each participant was encouraged to state one or more desired gender pronouns. On multiple occasions, Danielle expressed her gratitude for the rule that required participants to respect desired pronouns, regardless of visual appearance or passing ability. Her presence reminded others that visual cues provide limited and sometimes misleading information about gender identity.

Staff at clinics where I conducted site assessments often described cases of clients whose legal documentation listed them as 'male' and who alternated between overt visual presentation as women and standard men's attire. The consensus among clinic staff was that such individuals could be unhesitatingly addressed and treated as men, since these clients had neither asserted identities as women, nor corrected staff on pronoun usage. The staff sobered when I raised questions inspired by Danielle's presence in the group. Did these individuals wish to be considered women in the private confines of the clinical office, but to have their privacy preserved to safeguard their livelihoods, as in Danielle's case? Were they in the process of articulating a gender as women, bi-gender, or genderqueer while being unsure of how to explain their situation to staff or advocate for themselves? Were they trying to communicate their feelings and preferences passively or non-verbally? By examining these questions, we learned that consulting with clients and confirming their pronoun preferences is a vital first step in creating safe environments.

I was surprised to discover that many counsellors and clinic staff held the belief that their clients were 'regular people' (not of trans experience) unless

---

7 To be perceived as the gender with which one identifies; 'passing privilege' means being accorded the respect of acceptance as one's gender identity- this privilege is often taken for granted by people whose gender identities match their assigned genders, while being considered 'deception' in the context of 'trans' individuals. See Speer and Green, 2007 regarding the implications of 'passing' in psychiatric assessment. See Roen, 2002, for a discussion of debates on 'passing' within networks of individuals with non-assigned gender identities.

otherwise specified, an assumption that placed the burden of advocacy solely upon constituents. The fact that few staff had been exposed to people of non-assigned gender identities outside of media images exacerbated this problem. Women like Danielle, who did not fit the popular stereotype of the transsexual sex worker were often assumed to be 'transactivists', a mysterious single word utterance. These articulate and highly functional individuals were assumed to participate in an elusive and widespread network of others 'like themselves'. Many counsellors with whom I conversed were shocked to discover that many of our constituents were not activists; many of our support group members were not involved in any trans-related political action and many had never even met another person with an affirmed gender identity before attending the group. While the Internet does provide significant opportunities for interpersonal connection, many of our constituents either lacked home Internet access or were unable to gain the privacy required to engage in gender-related conversations online.

In Danielle's case, prior to the formation of our support group, she sought resources in multiple locations where she was unlikely to be recognised by people from her hometown. She told me that she had been rudely escorted from the women's changing facilities at an urban multi-service health centre on multiple occasions when she arrived for counselling sessions directly from her job as a manual labourer, and that she felt despondent about enduring counselling in an environment where she lacked the freedom to be herself. I wondered: Had the staff paid attention to when their clients' gender-related needs might change, and had they taken the initiative to enquire? Had they considered that their clients might have come directly from work on the occasions when they wore attire typically associated with men and therefore they were unable to wear women's clothing? Had anyone offered these clients the option of separate pronouns within the private confines of the exam and counselling rooms, regardless of whether they occasionally wore men's clothing? Had anyone provided options that might address the kinds of dilemmas faced by Danielle and others, rather than assuming that their lack of complaint ensured that their needs had been met adequately?

These questions barely skim the surface of the concerns that Danielle and those in similar situations needed their counsellors to address. To return to the question of why it is vital for counsellors to educate themselves about the intricate dynamics of people with affirmed gender identities, it is evident from the experiences that Danielle and others shared with me that without specific awareness of the situations faced by these individuals, even the most skilled therapist will be unable to provide quality care. A therapist should expect to expend some effort toward equality of service before these individuals perceive the same level of respect and feel the same level of comfort typically enjoyed by people with assigned gender identities (i.e. people whose gender identities match the ones they were assigned).

Pronoun Cueing and Mispronouning

The first person to assign a pronoun to another person in a social situation plays a pivotal role in establishing the person's gender identity and pronoun to those present. On a superficial level, pronoun usage may appear to be a social pleasantry that has little impact on service delivery. In fact, *pronoun cueing* is a fundamental component of social interactions that has the power to effectively challenge systemic inequities or to construct formidable access barriers.

Consider the case of Tara, a 19-year-old woman who did not 'pass' visually as female. After her domestic partner physically assaulted her, Tara was referred through several agencies. Based on both her visual appearance and identity documents that listed her as male, her caseworker at a human services programme consistently referred to her as 'he' while otherwise helpfully attempting to get her a bed at a local women's shelter. This *mispronouning* – usage of a pronoun that inaccurately depicted Tara's articulated gender identity – exacerbated the access barriers that she faced when attempting to access shelter resources. Staff at the women's shelter had difficulty understanding why someone referred to as 'he' needed to be housed in their women-only facility. Her caseworker was unable to advocate successfully for her with shelter staff that had a reputation (according to numerous affirmed women) of discriminating against them, in violation of local laws.

After being denied access, at least partly due to the incorrect pronoun cueing of her caseworker, Tara was placed in a mixed-gender homeless shelter. This shelter lacked the domestic violence services that Tara needed to cope with the domestic abuse that had caused her fresh bruises. Far more troubling was the fact that Tara, a young woman in crisis, was an easy target for bullying by men in the mixed shelter. Mere hours after surviving her partner's violent assault, Tara was sexually assaulted in the place she had gone for help. This time, her caseworker turned to a local organisation that focused on gay and lesbian clients. Despite their altruistic intentions, this organisation's staff had such a rudimentary grasp of 'trans' issues that their response to a traumatised, understandably suspicious Tara was to have her admitted to a psychiatric ward. While gay and lesbian clients served by this organisation had often reported positive experiences in this particular ward, which was known to have several nominally 'LGBT-friendly' clinicians on staff, women with Tara's gender history had disclosed overwhelmingly negative experiences with this unit to Lifelines. In Tara's case, while multiple factors contributed to the unfortunate outcome, mispronouning was a key element.

Many of the caring therapists whom I encountered were unaware of their intermittent pronoun slips until these slips were mentioned by me or by one of our constituents. While some therapists were embarrassed and troubled by their unintended errors, an alarming number of therapists initially attempted to justify this as client-specific, as a reflection on their client's level of success in appropriating the normative gendered behaviour of their non-assigned gender. One gay holistic mental health counsellor had the audacity to tell a client struggling to gain respect as a man that 'it's my psychic vibe telling me that I'm just not sure how deep this "being a man thing" really goes with you'. Another therapist told a constituent in the process of affirming his identity as a man that 'I only have trouble with your pronouns, because you don't really have guy mannerisms; my other clients seem more authentically male'. Counsellors attempting to justify or explain their mispronouning are misguided at best, destructive and counter-therapeutic at worst. It is important for therapists to remember that mispronouning is a form of verbal and psychological abuse. A wrong pronoun can wound as deeply as an ethnic or racial slur. The therapist has a moral obligation to be aware of this potential for injury and to make a concerted effort to avoid inflicting it. The emotional impact of mispronouning not only erodes a developing therapeutic relationship but also can have a dehumanising effect, as it denies recognition of the identity-related aspect of personhood and coerces the client into an ill-fitting gender straight-jacket.

Another common problem for people early in the process of *gender identity actualisation*[8] is the provider expectation that they would complain or notify the counsellor if the pronoun, given name, or gender identity that they were assigned did not work for them. During a site assessment at a local mental health clinic, staff assured me vehemently that none of their trans clients had ever objected to their system of colour-coding patient files by assigned gender category (rather than by affirmed gender identity). A crucial fact to consider is that silence does not automatically mean approval or comfort. At almost every one of our support group meetings, participants would describe situations in which they experienced discomfort with therapists and other service providers. In the vast majority of cases, they did not feel secure enough to voice their discomfort to the providers themselves. This was particularly noticeable among constituents who were in the first few years of affirming non-assigned gender identities and those from historically underserved ethnicities.

Many people in our group commenced the expression of their pronoun preferences tentatively, asserting that we could 'use whatever pronoun we wanted', claiming that they didn't mind. However, in almost all cases, after further conversation in which I – as facilitator – and other group members asked what they would *prefer*, these superficially ambivalent attendees expressed clear and unambiguous pronoun preferences. For counsellors who wish to support the gender affirmation process, this means taking the initiative to ask detailed follow-up questions designed to encourage clients who have not yet articulated the belief that they are entitled to their preferred pronouns. Many people in our group described the sentiment that they were inconveniencing others or making outlandish demands when explaining why they had chosen not to correct authority figures or friends who mispronounced them. For many of those who did not 'pass' visually based on normative stereotypes about gender in the dominant mainstream

---

8 A non-pathologising alternative to terms like 'gender transition' or 'sex change', *gender identity actualisation* (Vanderburgh, 2009) acknowledges that people who affirm their gender identities do not suddenly become a new gender, but instead actualise who they already know themselves to be.

culture, advocating for themselves in this manner felt belligerent and aggressive. While this kind of self-advocacy came more naturally to the minority of the group with backgrounds in activism, members of the group typically spent several meetings encouraging some participants before they felt liberated enough to accept our respect as their basic right.

The sense of liberation that the group provided for people initiating the process of gender identity actualisation was enhanced by the peer nature of our group. Yet this kind of life-affirming environment is one of the components of a safe, welcoming counselling relationship. By taking responsibility for asking detailed questions of clients, by offering a lavish banquet of choices rather than waiting for clients to pick the cheapest item on the menu (i.e., the pronouns and gender-associated name least likely to require effort or encounter resistance), counsellors demonstrate their willingness to take the journey of discovery with their clients, and to embrace new insights and the self-respect that is essential to thriving rather than merely surviving.

The need for providers to ask rather than to assume that lack of complaint translated into satisfaction was illustrated for one local clinician when he consulted with me on ways to help one of his long-term patients. A specialist in the field of communicable diseases, this caring provider had shared the joys and struggles of the Santiago family for five years. They had bonded closely during this time and seemed to have excellent communication.

When I spoke with Juan, my initial questions were about preferred pronouns and name. I knew from previous experience that I had to actively solicit this information by offering possible options in an encouraging and persistent manner. The first response was the predictable 'I don't want to inconvenience or challenge anyone' response I had heard from so many of our constituents: 'Whatever you want is fine', Then, after it was clear that I was sincere and willing to treat her requests seriously, 'Well, I sometimes go by "she", but it's okay to call me whatever you feel comfortable'. I persisted, 'What would be the *best* and most comfortable for *you*? Would you like me to call you by Juan or by another name?' In fact, after further conversation, it turned out that 'Juan' was actually Maria, whose experiences as a low income immigrant with limited employment background and difficulty expressing her emotions in English – despite her extensive practical vocabulary in daily life situations – made her hesitant to risk alienating her provider with what she considered might be, or might come across as, an ungrateful demand.

After five years of working with Maria's family, it had simply not occurred to her talented and responsive provider to investigate and solicit her pronoun preference and gender identity. It took fewer than five minutes for me to elicit this information from Maria during our initial phone conversation, because I knew which questions to ask and to pre-emptively address Maria's unspoken questions about how far I was willing to go toward taking her gender identity seriously. I found that this kind of advanced notification of provider attitude transforms the therapeutic relationship by meeting the client halfway in the communication process. Most people are not activists, and may simply be unable, unaccustomed, or unwilling to assert themselves before being provided with unsolicited supportive information from their providers. For many clients, gender identity affirmation may reveal itself in subtle hints and gestures, rather than in spoken form. One of the more widely praised counsellors among our support group members was appreciated for, in the words of one affirmed man, 'putting it all out there on the table for you as something on the menu before you even get up the courage to ask if you can add it in'. Maria's ability to get appropriate care improved as a result of sharing her information with her provider; the validation she received from her provider after he began treating her as a woman made her feel safe enough to disclose other details relevant to her wellbeing.

Even counsellors who express generally supportive attitudes toward trans youth may hinder their gender identity actualisation process by demonstrating less than full support for their affirmed genders with parents. For youth whose parents have not accepted their gender identities, counsellors have the potential to bridge parent-child communication gaps in their capacity as youth advocates. I was disappointed to discover that a counsellor working with vulnerable youth made the clinical judgement to use the name and pronouns with which the parent was most comfortable, rather than to use those asserted by Matthew, the 16-year-old affirmed man who was supposed to be her client. This counsellor mispronouned Matthew during our treatment team meetings and failed to use his preferred name and pronouns when he was not present, instead of setting an example of respect for other staff and Matthew's parents to emulate. Had this counsellor treated Matthew's gender identity as genuine and not a costume to be discarded at will when it was inconvenient or met resistance, his mother may well have felt motivated to consider offering similar acceptance.

From 'Gender Identity Disorder' to 'Gender Specialist Identity Disorder'

At a collaborative training for staff at a local hospital, Maria's provider commenced his presentation with an anecdote about the aforementioned experience, as a reminder to the medical and mental health specialists and department heads present that the best clinical training and experience in other areas do not necessarily prepare a provider to handle these kinds of situations effectively. The wisdom and humility of this realisation are crucial to providers who work with people of non-assigned gender identities. While providers who have significant experience with this population often take the presumptuous title of 'gender specialist' or 'gender expert', this grandiose nomenclature obscures the reality that there are as many gender identities, gender histories, and gender trajectories as there are individuals to claim them. One might easily become a celebrated 'gender specialist' or prolific author of 'gender therapy' guidelines, yet find oneself stumped when the responses that might have seemed beneficial and prudent in one case yield disastrous results in another. The 'gender specialist' mentality is dangerous because it presupposes a common link between people with affirmed gender identities, an ill-fitting set of blanket guidelines and prescriptions to govern something that is far less tangible and quantitatively structured than heart rate or body mass.

My position at Lifelines introduced me to people with gender identities that remain virtually unacknowledged in psychological texts, including genderqueer, kathoey, third gender, Two Spirit, agender, gender-free, bi-gender, tri-gender, androgyne, and macha, to name a few. Few providers are versed in counselling these individuals. As a result many people with gender identities outside the binary have difficulty finding appropriate psychotherapy, even from binary-gendered therapists of trans experience or therapists with extensive trans experience.

A transmasculine genderqueer individual whose assigned gender was that of a woman, Judah (who prefers male pronouns) shared his own challenges in seeking care:

> I was depressed when I graduated from college, probably because I had no idea what I was doing with my life and couldn't see any future for myself, so I went to get therapy. The first place I went was covered by my insurance and had some therapists. Just a luck of the draw kind of thing. I wanted to talk about how I had no friends and no direction and was miserable and what could I do? The therapist seemed fascinated mostly by my transmasculine gender, my relationship with my cross-dressing boyfriend, and other things of that nature. I left after one session because I felt like her entertainment – but I was supposed to be paying her! My next therapist was at (a popular clinic), which is supposed to know a lot about GLBT people, so I figured there was more of a chance she'd be cool. I mentioned my gender issues during my intake but also said I was not there for gender therapy. So I was assigned to a therapist who focused on helping me with my negative thoughts, increasing my self-esteem, finding a direction, and so on. It was great. But sometimes gender did become an issue, and at those times my new therapist became very confused. She would always point out when I contradicted myself instead of respecting that I had contradictory feelings, and no, it wasn't coherent and didn't make sense; why yes, I noticed that! I wanted a butch community but also sometimes wanted to transition (to being viewed as a man socially). Eventually I got frustrated with this because I felt that she just didn't understand me, so I left and went to a gender queer therapist someone else had recommended to me.

Unlike most genderqueer individuals who contacted me, Judah eventually managed to locate a counsellor who was both comfortable with and aware of his needs. Praising his genderqueer counsellor, Judah states:

> This therapist understands – and actually had first-hand experience regarding some aspects of – my gender experience. Ze^9 is able to acknowledge the

---

9   One of several 'third gender' English pronoun options (often used in conjunction with the gender neutral possessive pronoun 'hir') preferred by some genderqueer and non-binary-gendered individuals (See Bornstein, 1994, and Feinberg, 1998).

complexity and contradictions of my experience, to focus on gender when appropriate, or bring it in when it is relevant, without either ignoring it or making it the entire reason for all of my troubles.

The sensitivity that Judah's counsellor brings to their therapeutic relationship has translated into reduced access barriers. While most genderqueer individuals are unable to access hormones and surgery during gender identity actualisation, Judah's therapist assisted him in acquiring testosterone, something many 'gender specialists' routinely deny to people outside the binary. Since starting testosterone, Judah's self esteem and comfort with his body have increased significantly.

Counsellors are often stunned to learn that a high percentage of the unofficial provider complaints we received were about therapists who identified themselves as 'gender specialists', some of whom were among the most widely recognised names in the field. Since few of our constituents were willing to file official complaints, most of these concerns were addressed through cautionary anecdotes in our trainings or by advocacy meetings with individual providers. The rarity of formal complaints was an unfortunate consequence of the tremendous control that the widely used (though not, as many mistakenly believe, obligatory) *World Professional Association for Trans Health* (WPATH, formerly Harry Benjamin International 'Gender Dysphoria' [sic] Association [HBIGDA]) *Standards of Care* (Meyer et al., 2001)[10] gives to therapists of people seeking access to hormones and surgery related to gender identity, affirmation. These complaints ranged from simple disrespect to clear violations of client autonomy to ethical misconduct and abuse.

Consistently, the counsellors who garnered praise in our confidential support group, where attendees felt safe enough to warn against or recommend providers without fear of retaliation, were those who maintained modest perspectives about their 'gender expertise' and the needs of people with non-assigned gender identities. The few counsellors about whom I heard frequent praise were those who did not support the belief that people with affirmed gender identities had 'Gender Identity Disorder' (GID), who recognised the inequity of a system that forced 'trans' clients to jump through hoops to prove their validity in hopes of being accorded the same rights as other individuals, who understood the dangers of accepting the role of judge and jury in the psycho-medical gatekeeping system,

---

10   At this time, the 2001 WPATH guidelines are the most updated version available. While a newer version is imminently due for publication, it is worth noting that most clinics I encountered were still using outdated Standards of Care that dated as far back as the 1990s and few recognised the need to remain current. (See Lev, 2009 for recent recommendations for revisions to the current standard.) The contrast between updated standards and versions applied in clinical settings underscores the ethical obligation for authoring bodies to provide outreach and oversight to clinical settings that are ignorant of or resistant to employing the most recent standards.

and who forged therapeutic alliances with their clients to navigate the dictates of existing professional standards.

If trendy professional phrasing is considered necessary, the terms *gender advocate* and *gender affirmation counsellor* seem far more client centred and empowering. These terms emphasise the necessity for counsellors to address the extreme societal inequities facing people with non-assigned gender identities, while avoiding the hierarchical authoritarianism and arrogance of assuming the therapist as expert about something with which the client has far more intimate, daily experience. When I hear counsellors who market themselves as 'trans allies' make well-intentioned statements about the importance of clinical evaluation in determining whether someone 'really knows what they want', whether 'gender transition is right for them', whether the client is 'really transsexual' or 'should be allowed to get hormones or surgery', I wonder if they understand the paternalism and condescension of their approach.

While licensed therapists working within professional guidelines may often find themselves struggling to balance their ethical commitment to social justice with the dictates of a system that may inhibit this commitment, I still find myself surprised by the numbers of 'trans ally' therapists who do not engage in critical scrutiny of the institutional structures to which they contribute or of the discrepancy between giving lip service to client empowerment while simultaneously defending a system that undercuts client autonomy and self-actualisation. It is possible to work within the system without adopting its pathologising, dismissive mentality, as some fine strategic counsellors demonstrated in their conduct with our service recipients.

Dis-abling

I first learned about Jason's case from fellow trans activists when he was a teenager, years before we first met. An outgoing, active young man who was involved in various artistic, athletic, and community service activities, Jason had been trying to affirm his gender and obtain a prescription for testosterone for over six years. Several activists informed me that his numerous attempts had been consistently blocked through a combination of subtle manipulation and overt denials orchestrated by the host of providers who had 'cared' for him. The only counsellor who understood Jason and his needs well enough to give approval for him to begin 'T' (the vernacular term for testosterone commonly used by affirmed men) had stopped seeing him after questionable tactics by well-intentioned staff at a local organisation, who felt that he could not possibly know what he wanted. His large chest and high voice meant that he would be unable to pass visually as male in daily life without T. The discrimination Jason encountered was largely due to his having been diagnosed with a cognitive disability that accounted for his primary school reading level.

The moment I heard Jason's story from veteran activists, I vowed that if I were ever in a position to assist him, I would do so. I was delighted when Jason began attending our support group. I waited for him to share his experiences in the group before offering to help him speak effectively for himself with his providers, who had discounted his wishes in the past due to his inability to use collegiate language or grasp technical jargon. My desire was to give him a platform to express his needs by bridging communication gaps rather than speaking for him. Jason became despondent after watching his peers acquire hormones, while he had been seeking a prescription for years. By this time, I had booking privileges at the clinic of a local physician who had begun working collaboratively with Lifelines in some aspects of service provision. This physician was aware of the ease with which many people frustrated with rigid gatekeeping were able to obtain black market hormones and the perils to which that commerce exposed our constituents. He operated on a *harm reduction* standard that acknowledged the detrimental effect of service denial. As with other referrals, we exchanged disclosure of information forms from constituents, I briefed the physician on Jason's history, and I explained some of the access barriers that he had encountered due to his disability.

During the appointment, the physician patiently explained the informed consent document in language that Jason could understand, discussing sexuality, genital changes caused by testosterone, and other issues with admirable sensitivity. While Jason often found technical medical language daunting and unintelligible, this adept provider was able to translate the information into simple terms and check to make sure that Jason had grasped the message. Jason left the appointment with renewed hope and excitement about his future.

Unfortunately, within a few days, my voicemail was filled with intimidating, hostile messages from various professionals who had been working with Jason. Only one of these was a licensed provider, with whom I agreed to meet for conversation after exchanging the requisite disclosure forms from Jason. The others were from staff affiliated with a disability service agency charged with overseeing Jason's housing. It is relevant to note that Jason did not have a legal guardian and that he had the legal status of being mentally competent to make his own decisions about his care. One voicemail from a senior staff member at the service agency mispronounced Jason repeatedly, expressed alarm at the fact that he had been attending our support group, and contained vague threats about my being 'in trouble' for assisting Jason in affirming his gender identity.

I was unable to guess how inviting a vulnerable young man to attend a peer support group with others who shared some pivotal aspects of his history and needs was worthy of criticism. When I returned the phone call, the woman sputtered when I corrected her pronouns and used Jason's preferred name – a name that he legally made his official name years before he ever encountered this agency. I calmly explained the basics of gender affirmation to this woman and the fact that the physician and I were both in contact with his therapist. She seemed unable to articulate the source of her distress, resorting to repetitions of stock lines like 'but he has a *disability*!' – as if people with cognitive disabilities lack the ability to know their own gender identities or the human right to affirm that ability.

At our initial conversation, Jason's therapist was equally anxious. While she seemed far more aware of 'trans issues' and used the correct name and pronouns, she explained his trauma history and past suicidal ideation as definitive reasons why he should under no circumstances be permitted to access testosterone. She also expressed misinformation about numerous aspects of gender identity actualisation. As Jason was her first and only client of trans experience, she did not have past cases to challenge these inaccurate ideas. I explained that the denial of hormones to people with sexual abuse and trauma histories exacerbates their survivor issues by forcing them to continue having unwanted, intimate kinaesthetic experiences like menstruation or beard growth. Many of our group members had disclosed past genital mutilation and suicide attempts from the acute distress of this kind of kinaesthetic contrast. Several experienced physicians with whom I had presented had shared their insights about working with trans patients at our trainings, marvelling at the dramatic and sudden improvement in patient mental wellbeing caused by hormones alone, in the absence of any psychological therapeutic interventions. After describing these cases and explaining the distress that denial of T was causing to Jason, his therapist quickly became my ally in supporting him to get T.

Jason continued to face resistance and even derision from disability services employees who were afraid of his foray into a process about which they neither had nor desired basic knowledge. Yet despite these obstacles, he began to blossom after he acquired T. His therapist and even some of the staff who had been his detractors marvelled at his transformation – not the gender aspects, but the dramatic increase in his self esteem, confidence, and life satisfaction. Jason surprised many people by enrolling in courses at a local community college and obtaining assignment accommodations for his disability; the day he smiled and flashed his campus identification card at me to show that he had succeeded was one of the most rewarding moments of my life. After years of multiple psychiatric hospitalisations per year, Jason did not have a single hospitalisation after starting T.

At that moment, I recalled the agonising nights that I had lain awake replaying those hostile voicemails from ignorant staff in my head. What gave me the right to think that I knew best? These people were older and more experienced professionals than I, and in some cases had more extensive clinical training than I. Was I doing the right thing or leading Jason down a disastrous path with a catastrophic conclusion that everyone but me could see? As with many other complex moral dilemmas I faced during those three years, I sought the counsel of the retired marriage and family therapist who had agreed to be my clinical supervisor so that I could benefit from his wisdom and insight in just this kind of predicament. His response was characteristic of the astute perception that he graciously lent to our organisation. 'Gavi', he said in his quiet, compelling voice. 'You aren't the one making the decisions. It's not *your* decision to make any more than it is theirs. This is Jason's decision. Our only obligation is to support Jason in making *his own* decisions'. I realised that despite my moral convictions and ironclad resolve, the formidable pressure against my efforts to help Jason had caused even me to waver. I can only imagine how difficult it would be for an inexperienced counsellor or for someone in the same situation as Jason. Yet maintaining ethical integrity in response to institutional bullying and prejudice is one of the few effective ways to surmount these barriers. The therapist for whom the principle of client autonomy is foremost in the clinical judgement process is best poised to promote successful gender identity actualisation and prevent the potentially catastrophic impact of unwanted delays.

The Gatekeeping Industry and Standards of (Unequal) Care

Jason's case exemplifies the conflicts that can result when stakeholders in service professions feel that client needs threaten their livelihood or their authority. I discovered months later that at least part of the sentiment behind the intimidating phone calls stemmed from fear that Jason might move out of the programme's housing and services if their inability to address 'trans issues' was revealed, thus removing a lucrative source of income for the agency. As parties with financial, professional, and ego-based stakes in client outcomes, therapists must evaluate their motives very carefully when providing services or making clinical judgements. Whether therapists work for nationally funded public service agencies (like the NHS in the UK) or an international equivalent, private clinics, community health centres, or as independent providers, the fact that they receive a pay-cheque for their services is not a trivial detail. Therapists who defend their role as gatekeepers for access to hormones and surgeries related to gender identity actualisation may have consciously altruistic motives, but the severe risks inherent in playing judge and jury over whose gender identities are permitted actualisation and whose are deemed unauthorised outweigh the putative benefits.

My direct service experiences included hundreds of people who were harmed by well-meaning but misguided 'trans allies' and 'gender specialists' who blocked them from vital steps toward self actualisation. Several of the most widely used standards for dealing with trans clients seem to favour those who are financially independent, able-bodied, articulate, college educated, versed in theoretical jargon, and native speakers of the national languages in their countries. Even among therapists known for challenging racism, classism, ageism, ableism, sexism, heterosexism, and other forms of discrimination, these prejudices often emerged in their work with clients of trans experience.

DeShawn and Lakesha were among many Black-identified affirmed women who complained to me about being denied approval for hormones and surgery by non-Black counsellors of various ethnicities who considered them 'too masculine' to be women according to non-Black cultural gender norms. Lakesha's identity as a butch lesbian further challenged the prejudices of the therapeutic team that administered her mental health services, one of whom asked her during an evaluation meeting why she 'wanted to be a woman, when you can just be a straight man and have a normal dating life'. The fact that one of her providers was herself an out butch lesbian did not prevent the team from applying unequal standards to Lakesha; while her provider's status as an assigned woman apparently entitled her to deviate from normative straight femininity without endangering the legitimacy of her gender identity, Lakesha's butch lesbian identity was viewed as disqualifying her identity as a woman. The denial of medical resources to both DeShawn and Lakesha had severe negative repercussions that affected their abilities to gain legal employment, avoid police harassment, and access basic health care.

Similar discrimination delayed Hassan, an affirmed man whose penchant for wearing brightly coloured scarves and kohl eyeliner prompted his counsellor to speculate on the authenticity of his affirmed gender identity. Hassan was one of several affirmed men from Asian and Middle Eastern cultures who sought assistance from Lifelines in their efforts to obtain hormones or surgery, after having been informed by their therapists that they were considered unsuitable candidates because these affirmed men's traditional ethnic attire and cultural mannerisms read as 'feminine' or 'girly' to counsellors who lacked awareness of cultural differences in gender norms.

Professional assumptions about the appropriate ages for trans individuals to affirm their gender identities also clash with human actualities. One conventional paradigm classifies individuals as either 'primary or secondary transsexuals', with the latter referring to individuals who affirm their gender identities later in life. These 'secondary' trans individuals are depicted as having less authentic affirmed gender identities and less suitability for hormones and surgery. The underlying assumption is that a 'true' gender identity would have asserted itself at an earlier chronological age rather than after they had built families and functioned efficiently in their assigned genders. Marquetta's path to gender affirmation reveals the inherent classism and ethnocentrism of this notion.

An affirmed woman refugee from a Spanish-speaking nation, Marquetta had lived in her assigned gender as a man for decades, working 16-hour shifts in blistering heat during several decades as a migrant farm worker before she learned enough English to secure steady employment at a company that provided excellent retirement benefits. The eldest child in a large family, she was obligated to provide financial support for her younger siblings, and had limited educational opportunities. In her early 60s, Marquetta had only begun to have time and space to consider her own needs in the last few years and quickly realised that she wanted to affirm her gender as a woman. Although the decision to have genital and other surgeries has no bearing on the legitimacy of someone's gender identity, Marquetta chose to travel to Thailand for one of several possible genital surgeries as part of her gender identity actualisation process after she located a Thai surgeon who did not require therapist approval. Despite receiving full medical clearance that surgery was safe, she was denied approval by a therapist who considered her 'a poor candidate for surgery' due to the age at which she affirmed her gender. Prior to retirement, Marquetta lacked not only the financial resources to obtain surgery, but the time to contemplate matters beyond her material needs for basic subsistence. In this case, the only discernible difference between a 'primary' and 'secondary transsexual' was socioeconomic status and self-reflective leisure time associated with class privilege.

The many children and adolescents who sought assistance from Lifelines in their efforts toward gender identity actualisation were typically less fortunate than Marquetta, whose legal status as an adult gave her greater freedom to make decisions about her own body. It is comforting for those of us dedicated to our work as counsellors to dismiss examples of blatant discrimination encountered by DeShawn, Lakesha, Hassan, Jason, Marquetta, and countless others as mere 'exceptions', as atypical or as the fault of individual therapists. However, these inequities are a direct result of institutional discrimination enshrined in the *WPATH Standards of Care*. The unexamined assumption that only individuals with the social status to present pristine (and normative) textbook examples of 'genuine trans people' are worthy of the right to gender identity actualisation underlies many current policies and practises in psychological counselling.

The vast majority of the hundreds of people who either attended our support group or who contacted me individually for assistance shared horror stories of service denial and mistreatment by providers who insisted that they were merely following approved 'Standards of Care'. Many of these individuals – particularly those who were discriminated against in seeking hormones and surgery because of their non-binary gender identities – found ways to acquire hormones through unofficial channels in efforts at self-preservation that would not have been necessary if their providers had been actual rather than nominal allies. The most widely used versions of the 'Standards of Care' contain a 'Real Life Test' component. This 'Test' requires individuals to live 'full time' asserting their gender identity to the world prior to accessing gender affirmation-related surgeries that permit them to change sex markers on identity documents or use changing rooms at athletic facilities without trans-related harassment. Rigid provider adherence to these guidelines was directly responsible for severe physical safety hazards for our constituents.

Andrea, the desperate mother of a 17-year-old affirmed woman named Rochelle who used a wheelchair and suffered from chronic illness, was referred to me by her therapist after previous contacts failed to assist her. Andrea begged me to help her to save her daughter's life. They lived in a rural village where residents knew each other intimately, with little opportunity to maintain privacy or keep secrets. There were several counsellors in the village, but their connections with Andrea's employer and her church meant that she could not confide in them about Rochelle without risking her job or her social standing in the tiny community.

For several years, Rochelle had been desperate to obtain hormones or the fully reversible hormone blockers like Lupron Depot that prevent the trauma of 'the wrong puberty' in people under 16 years old. Unfortunately, due to extreme political backlash against some providers willing to assist people less than 18 years old with *kinaesthetic identity actualisation*,[11] all of the medical providers whom Andrea consulted adhered to rigid Standards of Care. These Standards required that Rochelle either undergo months of counselling or meet the aforementioned criteria known as the 'Real Life Test'.[12] Her physical condition made travel to a therapist's office precarious and her attempt at meeting the Real Life Test requirement was thwarted by a violent assault she experienced the first time she attempted to use the handicapped stall situated in the women's bathroom at her local community centre. Far from being an exception, Rochelle's predicament typified the unequal access caused by lingering inflexibilities in current Standards of Care.

On a weekly basis, I heard reports from affirmed men and women who were harassed and assaulted at banks, clubs, and routine traffic stops when presenting identity documents that did not match their visual appearance. One affirmed woman dropped out of a prestigious nursing programme after being repeatedly beaten in the face on her evening bus rides to and from classes. She had wanted to wait to live 'full time' as a woman until she could afford to move to a new city where people would not recognise her from her past public role as a man, but she was barred from getting surgery until she took this risk.

My past experience as a multilingual psychiatric caseworker prompted a local physician to refer an affirmed woman who had been unable to locate a counsellor fluent in her native language. Her patient Nasreen had a history of past suicide attempts that were prompted by her extensive trauma history. Concerned about the possible emotional fluctuations she might experience in the initial period of adjustment to oestrogen, Nasreen's health care team was unwilling to prescribe hormones without an agreement that she would attend regular counselling sessions to monitor her moods. At first glance, this safety precaution seems reasonable, prudent, and even requisite. Unfortunately, there were no counsellors who spoke her native language registered at the local centre and her providers had searched the entire region to no avail. She was seeing an English-speaking counsellor who was trying her best to meet her needs, while recognising that Nasreen didn't feel comfortable sharing the personal information required for psychological assessment with her counsellor due to their cultural and linguistic communication gaps.

Nasreen waited many months before we were able to locate a therapist who spoke her native language, during which time her well being deteriorated as a result of acute distress regarding the delay in acquiring hormones. Nasreen eventually decided to obtain hormones through unofficial channels, rather than continue to wait indefinitely. Any evaluation of the benefits and drawbacks of providing hormones to Nasreen given her history must also consider that blocking her access to a hormone prescription had a detrimental rather than neutral effect; in cases like

---

11   The process of acquiring hormones, hormone blockers, and various genital and secondary 'sex' characteristic-related surgeries to make one's embodiment match one's sense of self; often but not always part of the process of affirming one's gender identity.

12   For an ethical critique of these Standards of Care, see Hale, 2007. See Giordano, 2008, for an ethical critique focused on treatment protocols for adolescents.

Nasreen's, the medical dictate to 'Do No Harm' may provide compelling ethical justification for action.

Nasreen's situation illustrates the critical role that awareness and knowledge of a client's language and culture has in establishing therapeutic relationships. Simply being from the same cultural background or identity category as one's client does not in itself grant a counsellor a better ability to meet client needs; some clients of trans experience even found that trans therapists assumed far too much commonality or imposed their personal politics in unhelpful ways. Yet the frequency with which trans individuals from historically underserved ethnicities complained about analogous access barriers highlights one of the many flaws in placing therapists in gatekeeping roles. In addition, the combative nature of the gatekeeper-supplicant dynamic precludes the basic trust, respect, and encouragement of autonomy that are fundamental to therapeutic relationships.

The *WPATH/HBIGDA Standards of Care* may have become less stringent over the past two decades, but the popular requirement of either a 'Real Life Test' or several months of therapy is a formidable obstacle to many already marginalised people. Some people of trans experience who conduct provider trainings or who are employed by gender clinics defend the 'Real Life Test' as an essential and beneficial requirement before obtaining permission to access medical resources. Yet the suffering this requirement causes many disenfranchised individuals challenges the ethics of such an assertion.

When speaking with counsellors whose support for the current gatekeeping system and restrictive 'Standards of Care' stems from claims by trans presenters that these systems were helpful and necessary in their own gender affirmation journeys, I am quick to enquire about the backgrounds of these educators. With few exceptions, people with affirmed gender identities who support the current system have 'passing privilege', come from dominant cultural backgrounds, are above poverty level, are citizens by birth rather than immigrants, and/or do not have physical disabilities that would hinder travel to counselling appointments. Among these apologists, those who are employed at gender clinics and other gatekeeping institutions have a clear conflict of interest in the related debate, as their continued employment depends upon their willingness to abide by workplace policies. It seems disingenuous to use the existence of a few privileged trans individuals who defend and promote the current system as proof that the 'Real Life Test', specifically, and gatekeeping, generally, are beneficial and ethical, when the system continues to fail the most vulnerable among us. The therapist who wishes to avoid becoming an inadvertent oppressor should fearlessly interrogate *hir*[13]/her/ his relative resistance and compliance to gatekeeping within the scope of *hir*/her/ his professional practice.

---

13 A 'third gender' possessive pronoun preferred by some genderqueer and non-binary-gendered individuals.

Don't Drink the Alphabet Soup

The popular acronym 'LGBT' (lesbian, gay, bisexual, and transgender) conflates gender identity with sexual orientation and in so doing obscures LGB complicity in widespread discrimination and exclusion against people of trans experience.[14] The term 'queer' is often used interchangeably with 'LGBT' in counselling and outreach work, despite its divergent possible meanings. The uncritical inclusion of 'trans' in the 'LGBT' or 'queer' community umbrella masks the inequities faced by people with affirmed genders in 'LGBT' environments.[15]

Eric, an affirmed gay man who had donated hundreds of volunteer hours to a local queer organisation, expressed dismay when several fellow members of the organisation consistently mispronouned him at public venues. When Eric began passing as a man after several months on testosterone, he became increasingly frustrated with the inability of fellow volunteers to respect his affirmed name and gender pronouns. After several events hosted by this organisation during which his assigned gender was disclosed without his consent, Eric left the group and sought other social environments in the general community, where few people knew his history.

Negative experiences like those that Eric shared with me are regrettably commonplace in ostensibly LGBT environments. A shy affirmed woman in her mid-forties who had lived in her assigned gender until her recent birthday, Molly spent several weeks selecting an outfit to wear for her first time, wearing clothing that matched her style. Molly selected tailored blue jeans and a royal blue cardigan that accentuated her warm blue eyes. She pulled her hair into an elegant bun and added a hint of clear lip gloss. The style suited her modest personality and those of us from the support group who had chosen to accompany her to the café on this momentous occasion basked in the glow of her happiness as she began to relax and enjoy the evening. Shortly after she arrived, the evening took a decidedly unpleasant turn when several gay men from a local LGBT group arrived in drag and began taunting her for not looking 'feminine' enough. They insulted her hair, her outfit, and her lack of makeup before walking away to accost someone else. Frequent reports of equally hostile and ignorant behaviour against people with affirmed gender identities in nominally queer environments are of particular concern to me given the widespread tendency for social service agencies to refer individuals of trans experience to queer organisations with the assumption that these organisations are poised to meet their needs.

---

14   While some cultures and gender identities (i.e., kathoey in Thailand, kinnar in India, and Two-Spirit in North America) have historically integrated notions of sexual orientation and gender identity, the concept of 'LGBT communities' that is now internationally known and used in multiple languages has its roots in the emergent identity politics of mid-1960s civil rights struggles that informed AIDS activism in the wake of the 1980s HIV epidemic (Grover, 1991, p. 24).

15   See Weiss, 2004, for a discussion of this phenomenon in the US.

Affirmed men who identify as gay and affirmed women who identify as lesbian often face derision or disrespect in 'LGB' environments; some lesbian and gay 'community' events even bar trans participants from attendance. In addition, many of our constituents identified as straight or heterosexual in their affirmed genders. While some of these individuals identified as LGB allies and were regular participants in LGB-themed events, many others expressed reactions of alienation in response to what I term *coercive queering*, the act of automatically lumping people of trans experience into the category 'queer' without bothering to investigate accuracy or issues of consent. (This kind of 'trans as trope' mentality abounds in queer theory and gender studies.[16])

The aspiration of trans inclusion may prompt an increasing number of organisations to add what many trans activists consider tokenistic mention on their masthead, but the achievement of this goal is rare. As an incoming member of a regional task force that focused on 'LGBT', queer and questioning youth issues, I worked collaboratively with service providers to refine measurement tools for assessing 'LGBT' awareness in counselling and therapeutic settings. I quickly discovered that our printed materials mentioned 'transgender' but omitted any mention of trans-specific prejudice or discrimination. Instead, our materials stated the goal of challenging 'homophobia' to improve educational safety for 'LGBT' youth. The 'LGBT inclusion and awareness' assessment tool designed by the task force did not contain any mention of 'trans' aside from the ever-present 'LGBT' acronym.

Some aspects of the assessment tool reflected awkward attempts to take language and concepts popular in sexual orientation contexts and graft a letter 'T' onto them. The youth survey questionnaire contained the item 'have you been discriminated against for your LGBT sexuality?' inviting the question of why trans was being considered a 'sexuality' rather than a gender identity, gender expression, or process of gender affirmation. The architects of this document had also not considered the difficulty that a gay, lesbian, or bisexual respondent who was also of trans experience might face when answering this unintentionally convoluted question. Survey questionnaire items that dealt with 'coming out' demonstrated a similar lack of consideration for conceptual fit that made the 'T' seem even more haphazardly plastered onto the acronym.

The question 'to whom are you out about your sexual identity?' may have appeared straightforward to the authors. However, even if we overlook the fact that many trans individuals would bristle at having their gender assignment history considered a 'sexual identity', how would someone with an affirmed gender identity be expected to interpret the intent of this question? To whom are you

---

16   I have frequently attended 'queer' and 'LGBT' conferences where the only individuals of trans experience in attendance were the presenters, and these were seldom more than one or two individuals among dozens of speakers. Some colleagues of trans experience challenging inaccuracies in gender theories have even been publicly dismissed by gender theorists with assigned gender identities for 'not knowing enough about it'!

known as your affirmed gender? Who knows that your affirmed gender is not the same one you were previously assigned? 'Do you have images of LGBT reading materials clearly visible in your clinic waiting room?' one item asked. Usage of the acronym meant that clinics were able to respond affirmatively and rate as welcoming without necessarily having any trans-related material. The unexamined assumption evident from the wording of this question was that LGB inclusion automatically implies trans inclusion despite the fact that many of our service requests were from trans individuals who felt they had received unequal treatment at agencies with reputations for satisfying gay, lesbian, or bisexual services users with assigned gender identities.

This Alphabet Soup approach is prevalent in psychological research to such an extent that several task force therapists seeking statistics on trans youth had difficulty locating studies that even bothered to delineate trans from LGB and many of the citations they found used the four letter acronym despite their failure to include a single trans participant. In such a climate of erasure and invisibility, how can task forces and governmental bodies hope to develop policies that address the needs of trans youth adequately? The attainment of trans awareness and inclusion requires far more finesse than that evinced by a crude 'cut and paste' mentality.

Some nominally LGBT organisations attempt to remedy trans exclusion and ignorance by appointing people of trans experience to leadership positions. While integrating people with affirmed gender identities into management structures is an essential step toward the achievement of genuine inclusion, the logic behind this tokenistic manoeuvre configures an imagined and homogeneous 'Trans Community'. Predictably, these purported leaders are rarely selected from among the most disenfranchised and often gain acclaim in queer circles while simultaneously garnering negative reputations in trans only social networks for their complicity in the oppression of those whose backgrounds differ from their own. These externally or self-appointed authorities can become apologists for the gatekeeping system and for systemic inequities faced by less institutionally privileged trans individuals.

A trans educator who attended a town hall style meeting at a health conference with prominent providers was appalled by the efforts of several 'trans leaders' to impose restrictions against people under 18 seeking hormone blockers and hormone therapy. None of these purported trans leaders was a licensed medical provider or endocrinologist, yet their input might have contributed to increasing rather than decreasing access barriers for youth. These 'trans leaders' had not questioned their assigned gender identities prior to adulthood; they lacked personal experience with the intimate and constant violation of a puberty that clashed with their kinaesthetic identities.

If the Alphabet Soup approach is an ineffective and precarious method of challenging trans exclusion, counsellors may well ask which options exist for reducing exclusion and increasing awareness. The answer is that inclusion requires input from a multiplicity of perspectives, particularly from those whose extent of marginalisation precludes leadership roles. In specific instances, there may be strategic advantages to collective activism that integrates G, L, and B with T, while in other instances a kind of dilution effect seems to occur. For example, numerous 'LGBT' educators with limited presentation time choose to tack on cursory and superficial mention of 'T 'in the concluding five to ten minutes of a one hour presentation slot, rather than integrate substantive trans-related material throughout their presentations.

Organisations that include the 'T' should recognise that doing so is likely to increase the difficulty that current and future trans-led, trans-focused initiatives will face in securing funding, as LGB-based organisations tend to be more well-established, less politically controversial, and more palatable to mainstream donors. While many of the local organisations that focused on gay and lesbian concerns were able to gain funding for office space, their addition of the 'T' meant that Lifelines had difficulty securing local funding. During our efforts to secure financial assistance, my volunteers and I repeatedly heard from potential funders that other organisations 'had it covered' when it came to trans-related work, one negative consequence of the current trend for 'gay, lesbian, and bisexual' (GLB) organisations to add what many consider a tokenistic 'T' to their acronym. Unfortunately, these were also the same organisations that called us in – usually without paying us – to help them even begin to learn how to address the needs of their trans clients. Even in the provision of services, Lifelines staff and volunteers felt the disenfranchisement on an organisational level to which those of us with affirmed gender identities are subjected in our daily lives.

Beyond Cisgenderism

I have chosen to conclude rather than commence with a discussion of cisgenderism – and what it means for counselling psychology to move beyond it – because cisgenderist privilege and passing privilege typically render cisgenderism elusive in the absence of the concrete examples provided in this chapter. To restate the definition provided at the beginning of this chapter, my working definition classifies cisgenderism as the individual, social, or institutional attitudes, policies, and practises that assume people with non-assigned gender identities are inferior, 'unnatural' or disordered and which construct people with non-assigned gender identities as 'the effect to be explained'.[17] The 'everyday cisgenderism' encountered by Lifelines service users reflects a broader 'systemic cisgenderism'. Institutional and social systems are designed with the expectation that people needing to access them will match their assigned genders, and therefore provide services less effectively for people of trans experience. When we view psychotherapeutic and counselling practise through the lens of cisgenderism, questions emerge that allow us to challenge our beliefs and change our professional practice to bring it in line with our social justice values.

---

17   Hegarty and Pratto, 2001.

Far too often, counsellors and activists alike depict 'Trans People' as a cohesive demographic group, an 'Other' species that occupies a distinct social class and genus;[18] this portrayal condenses individual variations into oversimplified, formulaic notions that bear little resemblance to the lived experiences of thousands of individuals, morphing them into a conceptually cohesive theoretical unit presumed to share membership in some secret and mysterious 'community'. The assumption of 'community' among disenfranchised groups affects our ability to meet people's needs, since this generalised terminology swallows individual identities, as Jan Zita Grover explains:

> Whether used by spokespersons for (the gay community) or by its enemies, the people characterised as the *gay/homosexual community* are too diverse politically, economically, demographically to be described meaningfully by such a term. (One only has to attempt its opposite, *the heterosexual community* ... for the full absurdity of the term to become clear ...) ... the great diversity of humankind is reduced by means of the term to a single stereotype. (Grover, p. 24)

Grover's astute observation about 'the gay community' compels us to cease thinking and speaking of people with affirmed gender identities as a 'community' for similar reasons. While clusters of 'trans activists' in some regions may constitute a community, the vast majority of clients with affirmed genders are likely to fall outside this demographic. When we begin thinking of clients with non-assigned genders as individuals rather than as part of a homogeneous group, important questions will organically emerge from this realisation.

Consider the psychotherapeutic implications of cisgenderist language. Terms popular even among people of trans experience reinforce cisgenderist assumptions. For example, the term 'FTM', an acronym for 'female-to-male', reifies biological designations, placing a bureaucratic category as a salient element of identity and denies unqualified inclusion in an affirmed gender. 'Bioguy', a word used for assigned rather than affirmed men, contains the subtle implication that affirmed men are less authentically male due to a perceived lack of physical authenticity as male. The term 'gender variant' is problematic, because it assumes a social norm and vantage point from which to measure such variance: 'Variant' from what and according to whom? Even the term 'trans', used reluctantly throughout this chapter, is a norm-referencing descriptor that configures people with affirmed

---

18 The ideological assumption that people with non-assigned gender identities constitute a distinct class of person or homogeneous 'community' may be a form of Othering used to maintain or justify institutional cisgenderism, a strategic activist response to cisgenderism, or a form of internalised cisgenderism among people with non-assigned gender identities.

gender identities as 'the effect to be explained'.[19] While I have used 'affirmed man' and 'affirmed woman' for clarity, the need for the qualifier signifies the current climate of cisgenderism.

Notions of biology are inextricably bound up in concepts of gender identity in the field of psychology. Consider the current usage of 'gender' to refer to gender assignments, while the qualified term 'gender identity' is used to refer to the subjective sense of gender held by individuals. This usage reflects the ultimate subjugation of self-designated genders to the authoritative force of external gender designations in normative counselling ideologies. I have intentionally avoided discussing 'sex' because 'biological' sex designations involve taking a limited number of hundreds of biological dimensions, constructing two profiles based on these dimensions, and labelling the profiles 'male' and 'female'; the dominance of this taxonomy persists, despite extensive medical evidence documenting that many existing biological profiles do not fit neatly into either of these binary categories.[20]

In her critique of how academic psychologists' treatment of 'sex' as 'an ahistorical, pretheoretical notion' negates understandings of gender-associated embodiment and gender identities outside the binary, Mary Brown Parlee notes that trans activists 'have found it necessary to move beyond such bedrock concepts of common-sense and scientific discourses as "woman", "man", "female", "male" … simply in order to take into account the empirical variety of actual persons' embodied subjectivities'.[21] While Parlee's point may seem overly technical and unrelated to psychotherapy, it has relevance for counselling practise. Just as many people are born with biological profiles that do not neatly match 'male' or 'female', many people's gender identities do not graft onto their kinaesthetic identities in a normative manner. Take the example of Charlotte Karlsdotter, a Swedish affirmed woman with a beard who has been denied approval for surgery to give her a vagina[22] based on cisgenderist concepts about 'woman', 'man', 'female', and 'male'. While history contains numerous examples of bearded women, Charlotte has been discriminated against by providers who refused to consider the legitimacy of her embodied gender expression. Moving beyond cisgenderism in psychotherapeutic responses to Charlotte and others who transcend the bounds of scientific discourse means recognising their equal right to hormones and surgery for gender identity actualisation, thereby challenging the normativity project in

---

19   See Hegarty and Pratto, 2001 for an explanation of norms and 'the effect to be explained'.

20   See MacKenzie, Huntington and Gilmour, 2009, for one recent exploration of exclusion and forced normalisation of individuals who do not fit a 'male' or 'female' biological profile; while this study was limited to only a few participants, the authors provide useful historical background and raise important practical concerns, without constructing human biological variation as inherently pathological.

21   Parlee, 1996.

22   Volcano and Dahl, 2008.

which many 'gender specialists' are engaged. Confronting cisgenderism means asking our colleagues aloud why intersex babies' genitals are still being surgically altered at birth far below the age of informed consent, while women like Charlotte are routinely denied these surgeries.

Transcending cisgenderism means asking tough questions and initiating swift action, rather than becoming mired in theoretical discussions that exclude practical applications or evaluating policies without first having re-evaluated their problematic underlying conceptual frameworks. The terms that I have used are expendable; the critical enquiry behind them is not. Words like 'trans' and 'gender identity actualisation' are temporary placeholders to be replaced with newer concepts in the process of moving beyond 'cisgenderism' – another placeholder. For these reasons, instead of recommended reading, the endemic cisgenderism in psychology suggests that counsellors might be better served by recommended *thinking*, by seeking out new sources of knowledge production and new ways of viewing the world.

Challenging cisgenderism means more than being willing to switch pronouns depending upon whether you are alone with your client or addressing them in front of others, if they wish to keep their gender identity private. Moving beyond cisgenderism means more than merely providing clients with safe spaces to change and dress in clothing that reflects their gender identities. In the UK, eliminating the current requirement that service users seeking approval for hormones and surgery must 'dress in role' at clinical sessions would be a promising development for individuals facing Danielle's challenges; yet this improvement would do little to help those like Charlotte Karsdotter, whose ability to give informed consent would remain subjugated to normativity under current clinic policies.

Transcending cisgenderism involves recognising the counsellor's ethical responsibility to challenge injustice, the 'activism as therapy' approach advocated by therapist-activist Rupert Raj (Raj 2007). This 'therapeutic activism' is not a substitute for other forms of therapeutic services, but a complementary technique which frees space for therapists to address topics best suited to the therapeutic environment, including the creation of safe contexts for exploring the potential impact of medical and social gender affirmation decisions on employment, romantic relationships, parenting and child custody, and other major life domains. As many community psychologists have long argued, providing beneficial services to meet people's mental health needs is impossible unless their societal oppressions are confronted directly by clinicians.

In her recommendations for revisions to the 2001 WPATH SOC, therapist Arlene Istar Lev (2009) offers a responsible and humane approach to counselling people with non-assigned gender identities. Some elements of Lev's (2009) recommendations that seem particularly worthwhile are her explicit acknowledgement of the potential harm caused by mental health provider gatekeeping; her recognition of the need to develop harm-reduction approaches 'to assist marginalized populations in gaining access to trans-specific and general medical needs, regardless of whether they have been previously assessed using the SOC' (Lev, Table 1, p. 82); and her recommendation to 'remove the necessity to diagnose utilising the DSM ...', asserting that 'referral for medical services should not rely on meeting the diagnostic criteria of GID ...' (Lev, Table 1, p. 82).

Lev contends:

> ... The educated and informed transgender or transsexual client who is not suffering from mental illness or addiction, and is relatively stable socially and vocationally, and who has the support of loved ones, should be able to undergo a psychosocial assessment and referral process within a few sessions, typically between two and six hour-long appointments ... (Lev, p. 80)

While the revisions proposed by Lev would constitute a vast improvement to existing WPATH/HBIGDA SOC, these proposed criteria would still favour college-educated, financially secure clients with dominant culture ethnic and religious affiliations.

Lev follows this recommendation with a thoughtful discussion of the support counsellors should offer to individuals who do not meet the criteria excerpted above, such as those who have lost jobs or loved ones due to economic recession or disclosure of non-assigned gender identities; those with pre-existing mental health and self-harm issues unrelated to 'trans status'; or those who have developed psychiatric symptoms or addiction in response to past trauma or anti-trans brutality. When considering these support needs, it is vital for therapists to remember that denial of hormones and surgery often translates into denial of passing privilege; in the context of widespread employment discrimination and harassment of trans individuals in academic settings, failure to pass creates insurmountable barriers to vocational and financial stability for many individuals. For these reasons, while stability and sufficiency are clearly desirable for those in the midst of gender affirmation, requiring individuals to achieve vocational and financial stability prior to acquiring hormones may place them in an untenable predicament.

While some therapists routinely deny hormones to sexual abuse survivors who have not 'worked through their issues' beforehand, many Lifelines constituents like Jason found that they were unable to begin addressing their past trauma and truly thrive until they were liberated from the triggering and traumatic daily experience of existing in their bodies. Indeed, few among hundreds of Lifelines constituents met all of Lev's (2009) criteria, and many showed clear signs of relief from existing psychiatric symptoms and distress within weeks of starting hormones or acquiring surgery. It is axiomatic among trauma recovery professionals that genuine healing typically begins only after survivors are removed from abusive environments. The positive results of our constituents strongly suggest that the long-term process of trauma recovery may be aided significantly by providing hormones to some individuals, given that relief from the acute oppression of unwanted menstruation or beard growth may free emotional energy for vital recovery work.

While many Lifelines constituents who acquired hormones did not meet Lev's criteria, they did receive information about the medical and psychosocial risks and benefits of hormones from their medical providers sufficient to constitute 'informed consent' and those fortunate enough to have supportive therapists also discussed issues of disclosure management and social support with these therapists. Therefore, educational barriers and lack of family support may be issues for therapeutic discussion at the same time that acute needs for hormones or surgery are met, rather than automatic disqualifiers. When individuals share living space, parenting duties, or legal relationships like marriage or civil partnership, issues of disclosure become more complex and some interpretations of professional ethics may require client disclosure to spouses or parents; however, it is important to note that any ethical requirement for disclosure and spousal agreement should not be greater in this situation than in equivalent medical situations with major, irreversible consequences, as in the case of pregnancy or bariatric surgery.

Lev's (2009) assertion that clients may present with genuine mental health concerns unrelated to gender identity is an important one. Merely handing vulnerable clients a prescription for hormones out of a misguided notion that this 'magic bullet' will 'cure' their problems can be irresponsible and disastrous. The urgent need for hormones articulated by many clients must be accompanied by assistance that addresses their basic need for social support; subsistence level food and housing; freedom from domestic, workplace and public harassment and abuse; and opportunities for spiritual, intellectual, and creative growth. While several primary care providers from local community health clinics noted drastic reductions in psychiatric symptoms merely from the administration of hormones, independent of any other 'therapeutic' interventions (as occurred for both Jason and Judah), trans individuals often face greater risks of trauma-related concerns than those without the severe daily stress and abuse commonly reported by these individuals.[23] In many cases, assistance with acquiring hormones is insufficient to promote mental wellbeing in the absence of therapeutic support that addresses existing mental health concerns or the gender affirmation process itself- an ordeal that even those with substantial privilege and social resources often find daunting. Therefore, ethical practise requires therapists to explore which concerns are influenced by systemic inequities and therefore subject to improvement through activism, and which are best addressed through other therapeutic modalities; however, sometimes clients are the best judges of which modalities will work for them and therapy is not necessary or helpful for all individuals.

A therapist with an extensive background as an advocate on behalf of trans individuals, Lev's (2009) recommended revisions nevertheless fall within the scope of existing diagnostic frameworks rather than transcending the diagnostic lens. In an earlier piece, Lev herself raises ethical and practical concerns about the limitations of this lens:

---

23 For an examination of trauma among individuals with non-assigned gender identites, see Lev, 2004.

The utilization of GID to confer eligibility for gender variant people who need medical treatments serves as a confirmation that transsexual and transgender people are suffering from disorder and dysfunction and invites questions about the ability of the DSM to distinguish between mental illness and social non-conformity. If the person does not exhibit distress or dysfunction, are they therefore ineligible for treatments they are requesting? If the person exhibits significant distress and dysfunction are the then too unstable to receive treatment? What are the ethical implications of labeling gender variant people who are mentally sound with a psychiatric diagnosis to justify their receiving medical treatments? Can a diagnosis of a mental illness do anything but set the stage for protocols designed to repair a dysfunction? (Lev, p. 57)

These dilemmas and those addressed by Lev's (2009) recommendations exemplify the thorny issues encountered by therapists thrust into the role of gatekeepers. Given Lev's explicit caution regarding the tremendous damage therapists can cause through service delay or denial, coupled with the need for prudent deliberation to avoid the potential liability of licentiousness, one may question whether it is appropriate or ethical to place therapists in this vulnerable position with even more vulnerable clients.

Lev offers one possible solution to this dilemma within existing diagnostic frameworks:

An additional suggestion is to remove GID from the psychiatric nosology and use the already extant diagnosis of Transsexualism – described in the International Classification of Diseases, Tenth Edition (ICD-10), an Axis III medical condition – for medical treatments and reimbursement. The ICD diagnostic criteria would need to be revised and updated since they are based in a narrow view of transsexualism, but utilizing a diagnosis from a manual of physical ailments would validate the need for medical treatment without inferring a mental health diagnosis. Thus, gender transition would be an insurance reimbursable medical condition similar to pregnancy. Any mental health issues would be noted on Axis I or II as they would for any other psychological disorder, without mentioning the gender issues per se. A black person with anxiety disorder does not receive a racially identifying diagnosis, nor does a gay man with alcoholism receive a diagnosis highlighting his sexual orientation. This is not to say that race or sexual orientation do not impact anxiety or alcoholism, or even in some cases explain or justify these symptoms; it is not, however, part of the diagnostic label. (Lev, p. 59)

While Lev's suggestion is a viable solution that would drastically reduce pathologising of trans individuals and which is certainly among the most enlightened views within the diagnostic lens, her mention of pregnancy raises questions about the extent to which counsellors should be involved in assessment and evaluation of trans individuals when people seeking equally 'irreversible medical procedures' (e.g. surgical abortion, bariatric surgery, or designer labioplasty) with predictable psychosocial impact are not held to an equal standard of engagement with therapeutic counselling. To what extent does the assumption that service users seeking hormones and surgeries need therapeutic screening at all construct people of trans experience as a distinct class of person with diminished capacity for informed consent? How might counsellors react differently to assessment procedures that regulate medical access of other historically marginalised populations (e.g. women or indigenous populations) whose systemic oppression is addressed in an increasing number of counsellor training programmes?

Counsellors who balk at the notion that women seeking surgical abortions should be required to undergo pre-surgical counselling to 'make sure they are making the right decision' and 'really know what they want' (popular phrasings used by many self-styled 'gender specialists'), viewing the imposition of mental health assessment in the absence of overt psychiatric symptoms as a form of benevolent sexism,[24] seem hesitant to apply this discrimination lens to the treatment of trans individuals seeking hormones or surgery. Does the pervasive silence about paternalistic cisgenderism in normative counselling ideologies account for this discrepancy?

In her concluding remarks, Lev (2009) laments the current 'dearth of scientific evidence backing up much of the current SOC' (p. 95), stressing the need for 'evidence-based research' (ibid.) and 'SOC ... with substantial guidance in the treatment of complex clinical cases' (p. 82) including expanded discussion on 'issues related to assessment, treatment, and comorbid mental health issues' (ibid.). Yet the potential benefits of 'evidence-based research' are mediated by the manner in which the evidence is collected, the assumptions underlying the research methodology, and the ideological lens through which the research questions are formulated. Given the institutional cisgenderism endemic to normative counselling ideologies, 'evidence' that transcends the limitation of disciplinary prejudices and offers new insights to challenge pathologising or paternalistic views may prove elusive. Guidance regarding clinical treatment of complex cases may impose further rigidity on a system that already seems insular, rigid, and unresponsive to many service users. The ostensible neutrality of the term 'assessment' is counteracted by its linkage with 'treatment' and 'comorbidity' both terms that denote an underlying pathology or disorder; Lev's apparent objectives, to reduce pathologising of trans individuals solely on the basis of their non-assigned gender identities and to normalise trans experiences, are thwarted by the conflicting implications of these terms.

If one accepts the notion that therapists have a potentially appropriate function in the assessment process at all- that individuals of trans experience seeking medical resources should not be presumed mentally competent until proven

24   See Moya, Glick, Expósito, de Lemus and Hart, 2007, for a study of protective paternalism and the role of benevolent sexism in women's acceptance of protectively-justified restrictions.

otherwise (as is typically the case with individuals whose identities and expressions are socially normative) – one must grapple with the question of which training these therapists would require to provide helpful services. Curricula developed by those responsible for pathologising people with non-assigned gender identities may facilitate a decline in provider awareness, rather than serving its intended purpose. The 'substantial guidance' that Lev contends therapists desperately need is most likely to emerge when clients perceive themselves encouraged to give critical feedback to therapists and SOC-authoring bodies, without fear of retaliation or the expectation that their contributions will be dismissed. My work at Lifelines permitted me to engage in these kinds of dialogues with clinics and therapists and to ensure that our constituents felt comfortable contributing their experiences to training curricula. Yet I frequently hear from service users at 'gender specialist' settings that they are too concerned about service denial or negative repercussions to launch formal complaints. As long as professional guidance remains disconnected from this essential client feedback on the outcomes of its application, training programmes will fail to provide meaningful insights for mental health clinicians.

A local counsellor of trans experience who was held in high regard by many of our support group participants told me that the most valuable insight she gained from her professional training was the view of therapy as 'a form of social justice activism that empowers disenfranchised people to tell their own stories rather than having others speak for them'. The 'telling' may take the form of words, while others may 'speak' through activism, dance, or various forms of radical theatre that enable individuals of all literacy levels to share and transcend oppression.[25] To reach beyond cisgenderism, we must move beyond the confines of the counselling session into the institutions and professional associations within which we practise, and gain an intimate understanding of the systems that impact our clients' lives. In addition to offering new 'transpositive' therapeutic models like the aforementioned approaches by Raj (2007) and Vanderburgh (2009) (both experienced therapists with non-assigned gender identities), Lev's (2004) narrative approach, or Fraser's (2009) depth psychotherapy practise, counsellors should examine the culturally-specific assumptions of the 50-minute talk therapy model and be willing to offer non-verbal or solitary formats (i.e. meditation or home yoga) that match client needs.

Many experiences were omitted from this piece. These tableaus are intended to provide only rudimentary foundations for transcending cisgenderism. If these abridged portraits have demonstrated the nuances and intricacy of providing counselling that both challenges cisgenderism and transcends it; if you are motivated to confront cherished professional convictions and to interrogate your clinical judgements rather than to adhere perfunctorily to guidelines that promote normativity; if you are moved to critically evaluate the unexamined assumptions that underlie your counselling ideology, then I urge you to join the small but

---

25   For information about the usage of theatre as a therapeutic modality and/or as a form of client empowerment, see Boal, 1995, and other work by Augusto Boal.

dedicated ranks of your fellow counsellors who are dedicated to advancing the psychological wellbeing, autonomy, and equal rights of people with non-assigned gender identities.

Acknowledgements

My sincere thanks to editor Lyndsey Moon for her patience and support; to Gay Bradshaw, Toni Brennan, Elias, Martha Ferrito, Jackie Goss, Caroline Kersten, Tucker Lieberman, Danielle Maxon, Michelle McGrath, Jesse Pack, T. Plowman, Céline Rojon, and Bree Westphal for input on previous drafts; to 'Judah' for permission to print his narrative; to Sruli Beren for being spirit kin and inspiration; to my academic supervisor and mentor Peter Hegarty for everything; to Carla Garrity for believing in me; to Adrian Coyle for polishing my critical analytic skills in MSc assignment feedback; to therapist Arlene Istar Lev for her constructive critical feedback, encouragement, and collegial dialogue; to clinical supervisor Brian Kovacs for helping me to find and scrutinise my moral compass; to Tim Cavanaugh for opening the very first medical door; to all of the Lifelines constituents, service providers, volunteers, board members, and supporters whose perspectives and experiences informed this chapter; to anyone whom I have unintentionally omitted here; and most of all to Brenna McReynolds and Victor Ellingsen, for carrying the torch. I pray that I have done all of you justice.

References

Boal, A. (1995), *The Rainbow of Desire: The Boal Method of Theatre and Therapy* (London: Routledge).

Bornstein K. (1994), *Gender Outlaw: On Men, Women and the Rest of Us* (New York, NY: Routledge).

Buijs, C. (1996), 'A New Perspective on an Old Topic' (soc.support.transgendered newsgroup), 16 April.

Feinberg, L. (1998), *Trans Liberation: Beyond Pink or Blue* (Boston, MA: Beacon Press).

Fraser, L. (2009), 'Depth psychotherapy with transgender people', *Sexual and Relationship Therapy* 24: 2, 126–142.

Giordano, S. (2008), 'Lives in a chiaroscuro. Should we suspend the puberty of children with gender identity disorder?', *Journal of Medical Ethics* 34: 8, 580–584.

Grover, J.Z. (1991, 3rd reprint), 'AIDS: Keywords', in Crimp, D. (ed.), *AIDS: Cultural Analysis/Cultural Activism* (Cambridge: MIT Press).

Hale, C. J. (2007), 'Ethical problems with the mental health evaluation standards of care for adult gender variant prospective patients', *Perspectives in Biology and Medicine* 50: 4, 491–505.

Hegarty, P. and Pratto, F. (2001), 'The effects of social category norms and stereotypes on explanations for intergroup differences', *Journal of Personality and Social Psychology* 80: 5, 723–735.

Lev, A. (2004), *Transgender emergence: Therapeutic guidelines for working with gender-variant people and their families* (Binghamton, NY: Haworth Clinical Practice Press).

Lev, A. (2005), 'Disordering gender identity: Gender identity disorder in the DSM-IV-TR', *The Journal of Psychology and Human Sexuality* 17: 3–4, 35–69.

Lev, A. (2009), 'The ten tasks of the mental health provider: Recommendations for revision of the world professional association for transgender health's standards of care', *International Journal of Transgenderism* 11: 2, 74–99.

MacKenzie, D., Huntington, A. and Gilmour, J. (2009), 'The experiences of people with an intersex condition: A journey from silence to voice', *Journal of Clinical Nursing* 18: 12, 1775–1783.

Meyer, W., Bockting, W., Cohen-Kettenis, P., Coleman, E., DiCeglie, D., Devor, H., Gooren, L., Hage, J., Kirk, S., Kuiper, B., Laub, D., Lawrence, A., Menard, Y., Patton, J., Schaefer, L., Webb, A. and Wheeler, C. (2001), 'The Harry Benjamin International Gender Dysphoria Association's standards of care for gender identity disorders, sixth version', *International Journal of Transgenderism* 5: 1.

Parlee, M. (1996), 'Situated knowledges of personal embodiment: Transgender activists' and psychological theorists' perspectives on "sex" and "gender"', *Theory and Psychology* 6: 4, 625–645.

Raj, R. (2007), 'Transactivism as therapy: A client self-empowerment model linking personal and social agency', *Journal of Gay and Lesbian Psychotherapy* 11: 3, 77–98.

Roen, K. (2002), "Either/or' and 'both/neither': Discursive tensions in transgender politics', *Signs* 27: 2, 501–522.

Serano, J. (2007), *Whipping Girl: A Transsexual Woman on Sexism and the Scapegoating of Femininity* (Seattle: Seal Press).

Speer, S. and Green, R. (2007), 'On passing: The interactional organization of appearance attributions in the psychiatric assessment of transsexual patients', in *Out in Psychology: Lesbian, Gay, Bisexual, Trans and Queer Perspectives* (New York: John Wiley & Sons Ltd.), pp. 335–368.

Vanderburgh, R. (2009), 'Appropriate therapeutic care for families with pre-pubescent transgender/gender-dissonant children', *Child and Adolescent Social Work Journal* 26: 2, 135–154.

Volcano, D.L. and Dahl, U. (2008), *Femmes of Power: Exploding Queer Femininities* (London: Serpent's Tail).

Weiss, J.T. (2004) 'GL vs. BT: The archaeology of biphobia and transphobia in the U.S. lesbian and gay community', *Journal of Bisexuality* 3, 25–55.

Chapter 10

Azima ila Hayati – An Invitation in to My Life: Narrative Conversations about Sexual Identity

Sekneh Beckett

In recent years, I have made it clear in public settings that, as a psychologist from a Muslim background, I am most willing to speak with Muslims who are negotiating their sexual identities. At the same time, I have become known to the local queer community.

These two factors have meant that I have found myself in conversations with people of Muslim heritage about sexual identity, which I very much enjoy. My passion for hearing the stories of Muslims who are negotiating their sexual identity increased recently, when I learnt of attempts within the field of Islamic psychology to work in collaboration with Christians in order to 'rehabilitate gays and lesbians'. Within professional discussions, I have heard statements such as: 'You must know that the punishment for homosexuality is to be stoned to death, and that the body of a homosexual person must be cremated because they are diseased. We must save them'.

Games of Truth

When listening to these sorts of views about homosexuality, I have noticed that these thoughts within any community become a 'game of truth'. This term was coined by Foucault to refer to the function of thought and its specific practices. Foucault defined such a 'game' as 'a set of rules by which truth is produced' (2003a, 38). He further proposed that these 'games of truth' have real effects on people's lives:

> In a given game of truth it is always possible to discover something different and to more or less modify this ... (2003a, 39)

Foucault's interest in exploring the manifestations of truth games, and their relationship with power, is highlighted by his use of the example of medical institutions. He deconstructs the historical, social, and economic contexts that legitimised the prescription of medical labels to individuals presumed to be 'mad'.

His argument is not designed to debate the therapeutic effectiveness of medical approaches, nor to invalidate them. He further states that he is not saying madness does not exist, but questions the political birth of the concept and seeks to make transparent the discourses at play within the field of medicine.

Making discourses transparent 'renders visible' games of truth and power. In turn, this exposes the practices embedded in the socio-political contexts that support these truths, and opens space to discover something different (2003a). Let me now try to apply this approach to the experience of young queer Muslims. What would it mean if a young person of the Islamic faith wanted to consult with a health professional about their sexuality and they received information that there is a service to rehabilitate them? What might be the effects of such messages when lesbian and gay youth are at elevated risk of suicide attempts, and that the mean age of suicide attempts precedes coming out and first same-gender sexual experience? (Nicholas and Howard, 1998). What might be some of the 'games of truth' for people of Muslim heritage who identify as homosexuals? How might I be able to engage in conversations that honour their religion, while at the same time exploring different identities that might not fit with religious scriptures? These questions have shaped my exploration of the complex realms of religious identification and sexuality.

Queerying the Concept of 'Coming Out'

Not only are there 'games of truth' within the Muslim community, but also within queer communities. One such 'game of truth' relates to the thought and practices associated with 'coming out'. The following reflections have been influenced by conversations I have had with people who identify as Muslim queers about the isolation they have experienced when in contact with 'mainstream' gay, lesbian, bisexual, transgender, intersex, queer, and questioning (GLBTIQ) services. The Gay and Lesbian Counselling and Community Services of Australia define 'coming out' as 'telling someone you are lesbian or gay? Someone who has not come out is referred to as being 'in the closet' (Gay and Lesbian Counselling and Community Services of Australia, n.d.). At times within the queer community, assumptions are made that in order to live a 'truly gay or queer life' it is necessary to 'come out' in certain ways.

The complexity of this idea has been highlighted by the historian Shannon Woodcock (2004, 2). Woodcock identifies as an 'Australian ethnic woman who desires women'. Her paper discusses the globalisation of the same-sex politics and the queer rights movement. She states that the political form of identification associated with 'coming out' in the West positions itself in the binary of homosexuality and heterosexuality, and this poses a problem:

> It is vital to examine how western discourse of freeing LGBT individuals from repressed social positions through political action primarily requires local

subjects who answer to those very specific names of lesbian, gay, bisexual and transgender ... (and yet) there have always existed communities that identify through same sex practices in eastern Europe, and these communities have performed their identities in a variety of ways, in a variety of social spaces. I argue that Romanian and Albanian women who desire women have had a detailed, dynamic and beautiful system of strategies for identifying themselves and others, and that the western project of developing LGBT communities attempts to contain this strategic dynamism.

In her analysis, Woodcock questions whether this containment 'masquerades as salvation', and refers to Hoad who claims that:

> ... to assert the universality of a specific historical agent can, and arguably is, closing down spaces for these participants without replicating the set of historical circumstances which allowed gayness to have historical agency in the west. The universality that promises liberation ends up as oppression. (Woodcock, 2004, 2)

Woodcock interviewed women from Albania and Romania who had only experienced relationships with women and yet disclosed their discomfort with the 'western pressure to identify as lesbian'. While acknowledging the importance of coming out in creating a sense of community, and to support others who have come out, Woodcock explains that the idea of coming out for the 'desire for lesbians to become more visible is itself an incitement to discourse' (2004, 8). Seen in this light, within western discourse, individuals are encouraged to come out and confess their sexual identity 'which in turn creates a new set of organising sexual identities which damage existing, more subtle, networks of communication of sexualities and identities' (Woodcock, 2004, 11).

On the other hand, Irshad Manji (2003, 216), an author who identifies as a lesbian Muslim, 'thanks God for the West'. She testifies that 'the spirit of exploration' in the west is 'oxygen' for which she is grateful. She writes: 'In much of North America, Muslims have the freedom to be multi-dimensional ... Pluralism of people, pluralism of ideas, draw the connection. I did, and that connection has so far saved my faith in Islam'.

As I ponder on these ideas, I notice the many complexities and contradictions they contain. One might argue that, if it was not for the process of coming out and the queer communities this has created, we might not have the liberties or the language with which to write about this topic. In response, it seems appropriate to state that my curiosity is guided by Foucault's (2003b, 172) interview entitled 'So is it important to think?'. Within this interview he states:

> A critique does not consist in saying things aren't good the way they are. It consists in seeing on what type of assumptions, of familiar notions; of established unexamined ways of thinking the accepted practices are based.

The work done in the field of supporting and developing GLBTIQ communities has been invaluable, and the concept of 'coming out' has played an important part in this. I acknowledge the importance of coming out as a community concept. It has given voice to the ongoing struggles to attain legal recognition and support services for the GLBTIQ communities, and played a significant role in rendering visible the human rights issues. I also wish to acknowledge that many queer groups take great care in leaving any decisions about 'coming out' to the person concerned (see, again, Gay and Lesbian Counselling and Community Services of Australia, n.d.).

Despite this, for some, including some young queer Muslims, the discourse associated with 'coming out' can be fraught. It has been my honour to witness alternative ways in which some queer young people define their existence and identifications. It has been these experiences that have led me to write this paper.

The Idea of 'Coming In'

In my therapeutic work, I have arrived at these points of reflection: How do we give thought and voice to people who might experience being marginalised *within* the marginalised groups in society? What happens when certain practices do not speak to all members of the group? How can we, as counsellors, free ourselves from prescribed ideas about 'identity acceptance' and open ourselves to learn something new, something different?

In light of the above ideas, and after many conversations with my brother, we coined the term 'coming in'. This term refers to the conscious and selective invitation of people into one's 'club of life' (White, 2000). Although it might be a matter of semantics, I have found it an experience-near definition that has opened space for many queer Muslim people with whom I consult. The way the concept works is illustrated in a transcript later in this article.

Acts of Resistance

I hold a strong fascination in therapeutic encounters for uncovering thoughts and actions of protest and resistance (White, 1995; White and Epston, 1990). This opens the possibility to notice that ... in power relations there is necessarily the possibility of resistance because if there was no possibility of resistance ... there would be no power relations at all ... if there are relations of power in every social field, this is because there is freedom everywhere (Foucault, 2003a, 34–35).

With this in mind, my intention within therapy is to explore the art of resistance and to research and honour these creative acts. This idea is reinforced by the humorous, yet poignant Ethiopian proverb (cited by Wade, 1997): 'when the grand lord passes, the wise peasant bows deeply and silently farts'. This proverb has been a source of laughter when I have shared it with people I consult, and I have sometimes asked: 'Has there been a time when you have done the silent fart when the grand lord passed?' This highlights the relationship between oppression and creative acts of resistance (Mears, 2002). I am always curious about researching the presence of resistance in people's lives.

Uncertainty

Jamil is a young Muslim Arab gay man who was referred to me by a local queer support group. Jamil told me that he wanted to explore the concept of 'coming out', and the difficulties some assumptions about this concept had caused for him. A process of deconstructing the concept of 'coming out' supported him to research alternative ways of defining his journey, ways that accommodated to his lifestyle and preferences. These are described later in this paper. Yet Jamil was experiencing ongoing tension with his brother, Hassan, who holds strongly to his Islamic faith and was experiencing difficulty accepting his brother's sexuality. Jamil told me that he wanted Hassan to join our therapeutic conversations as an outsider witness (Russell and Carey, 2004; White, 2000).

Initially, I was in doubt about whether this would be a helpful experience or even whether Hassan would be willing to join us. I engaged in some thought about this and reflected on the following questions: How do I orientate myself to take a position of interest and discovery given homophobic ideas might be presented? If I hold a certain attitude towards people who hold homophobic ideas, how might I be entering into 'games of truth'?

In taking a position to embrace the idea that 'there is no certainty, only degrees of uncertainty' in therapeutic encounters (Amundson, Stewart and Valentine, 1993, 120), I prepared to meet with Jamil and Hassan. Two key concepts informed how I approached this conversation. The first involved a determination to explore, research, and honour Jamil's resistance to homophobic attitudes. The second involved thinking through my responsibilities to scaffold the conversations in particular ways.

Scaffolding Conversations – The Architecture of Possibilities

In my conversation with Jamil and Hassan, I hoped to assist these brothers to move from what was 'known and familiar' about their relationship (which had been characterised by conflict around Jamil's sexual identity) towards what might be 'possible for them to know'. When people consult therapists, it is often because they are telling stories about their lives and relationships that are stuck within the realm of the known and familiar. As therapists we have the responsibility to scaffold conversations to progressively and incrementally support specific learning tasks, and to facilitate movement towards what is possible for people to know about their lives. This, in turn, creates new options for action. Providing this scaffolding is akin to providing an architecture of possibility.

White (2006) in reviewing the ideas of Vygotsky, a developmental and learning theorist, states that learning is the product of social collaboration and that it is through interactions with significant others that people can explore what they might be able to accomplish in life. Therapeutically, White (2006) asserts that the therapist is required to effectively scaffold conversations to support people to incrementally and progressively distance from the known and familiar issues that affect their lives. This space in turn provides the foundation for people to develop a sense of personal agency and to start influencing the design of their own life. The gap between the 'known and familiar' and 'what is possible to know' was described by Vygotsky (1986: 86) as the 'zone of proximal development'. Navigating this zone occurs through social collaboration, through scaffolded conversations, and with the audience of significant others.

During therapeutic conversations with Jamil, we tried to identify and expose the 'truth games' that supported the dominant story. Through this process, we began to traverse the gap between 'the known and familiar' and 'what is possible to know'.

Jamil started to talk about the ways in which he responds to these 'truth games' and to reflect upon how he has come to value his life and identity. The five categories of scaffolding described by White (2006), which can shape therapeutic conversations, influenced the questions that I asked:

Distancing task (from the known and familiar):	Therapist's task is to:	Sample questions include:
Low-level	Characterise specific objects and events	Can I get to know the issue a little better and events by asking some questions? What name, characteristic, or words might you give to describe this issue?
Medium-level	Bring into relationship specific world in order to develop chains of association	Can you tell me when you first started objects and events of the person's to notice this issue? Has it changed over time? Have you noticed what might be happening at those times?
Medium high-level	Reflect on these chains of associations	What influences has this had on the of associations way that you see yourself? What effects does it have on your relationship with ...? What do you think about this?

High-level	Abstract learning from the concrete and specific circumstances to form concepts about life and identity	When this is present, how does it get in the way of your hopes and dreams? What does this knowledge say about what you value in life, about what is important to you? Can you tell me a small story about a time when these values have played a role in your life?
Very high-level	Formulate a prediction about the outcome of a specific action founded on this concept development, and encourage the planning for and initiation of such actions	If you were to act in accordance with this value, what steps might you take? Who might support you in this journey? How?

These ideas provided the foundation for my conversations with Jamil. The first step was to deconstruct with Jamil many of the taken-for-granted assumptions about life that had led to negative effects on his life. The second step was to ask questions that honoured and acknowledged Jamil's journey in navigating his sexual, cultural, and religious identities.

The process of venturing from the 'known and familiar' to what was 'possible to know' involved engaging in a definitional ceremony (Myerhoff, 1982; White, 2000) with Jamil and his brother Hassan. In accordance with the definitional ceremony process, in the first stage of the ceremony Jamil shared the stories of his life before an outsider witness, his brother Hassan. In the second stage of the ceremony, Hassan was given the opportunity to respond by re-telling certain aspects of what he had been an audience to. These re-tellings were shaped by specific traditions of acknowledgement (White, 2000).

Jamil's Story

Jamil is a 24-year-old Australian-born Lebanese Muslim man who told me that he had 'identified as gay from the day I was born'. He was referred to me by a colleague from the local GLBTIQ organisation. During our meetings, Jamil engaged in conversations about the importance of unpacking the games of truth, naming various acts of resistance, and developing a process of inviting certain family members into his life. Jamil still resides at his parent's residence with his unmarried siblings. He informed me that in his family 'it's not a common practice to move out of home until we get married'. I was also informed that his relationship with his eldest brother, Hassan, aged 26, had been volatile since they were very young. I experienced this volatility when Hassan contacted me and said that I needed to 'help his brother' by endorsing the Islamic scriptures, and to 'stop reinforcing his sexuality'. When I shared the importance of my ethical position, one that is informed by the narrative ideas of curiosity and support, he hung up.

Later that year, I received another call from Hassan telling me that he had 'f— ed up'. When I said I didn't quite understand what that meant, he said, 'I tried to slap some sense into Jamil … his tears killed me … I know it's not his fault'. I took the opportunity over the phone to ask Hassan some questions about the slapping, its effects on the sort of relationship Hassan wanted to have with his brother, and how he had got disconnected from his better judgement. He said to me, 'Why don't you get it? Aren't you a Leb? Aren't you from a Muslim family?' I contacted Jamil to ascertain his safety and we talked about Hassan's surprising phone call. Jamil laughed and said that he knew that it would be handy to leave my number on the fridge in case other members of the family needed it! I discussed the possibility of inviting Hassan to our next session so that we could involve him in a definitional ceremony. Jamil said that he would invite Hassan, but was not hopeful that he would accept the offer. As it turned out, Hassan took up the invitation.

When he turned up to our next meeting, greeting him and acknowledging him was religiously sensitive. Out of respect, I did not offer to shake his hand, and did not hold eye contact. I talked at length about the definitional ceremony structure, and how this would provide a foundation for us to work together. The room was organised so that initially Jamil and I sat facing each other in the centre of the room, with Hassan behind his brother in an audience position to the conversation. It was important for me, given the potential precariousness of the situation, to be transparent about my ethical obligation to contact relevant services if I thought personal safety or the safety of others was compromised. In order to establish further safety and rapport, I asked them: 'If any of the following questions take you to a place that you do not feel comfortable, or perhaps you don't want to answer, could you please alert me to this? How might you do that?' These preparatory steps set a foundation for the conversation that followed. I have included some of the transcript from this conversation here:

Jamil, Why is it important to you for your brother to join with us today?

I want us to get along. I know that he doesn't get me being gay, but I hope if he listens to us talk he can understand. If we are at home I don't get the chance to tell him about my life. We just bicker and bicker. I hope he can hear me because I want to be close. We are family. I want him to know how tough it is to be gay, Arab, and Muslim.

Jamil, I'm interested in hearing more of your thoughts about the relationship between being gay and being from an Arabic-speaking and Muslim background?

It's not something you would wish on your own enemy – to be Muslim and homosexual in today's climate – oh yeah, and an Arab. Think about it. In some Muslim nations based on interpretations of the Quran, the killing of gays and lesbians is enforced. Then there is a belief that homosexuality doesn't exist in the Arab world; that it's a disease of the West and it's only the weak that get contaminated.

We have spoken before about how some of these beliefs and ideas are like 'games of truth'. What might be some of the 'games of truth' played out in society?

Well the games of truth are more like what the politicians and religious leaders use to gain power. Every move they make they try and take a piece of you.

Can you tell me more about what you mean by that?

Well, just today, the Premier of this state has made unfavourable comments about a childcare centre because they read a book to the children there that features a little boy with two fathers. I think this book, *The Rainbow Cubby House*, is a great book, but people have argued about it in the media saying that kids shouldn't get involved in 'gay issues'. Some critics, including my family members, are saying that kids don't need to know about gay sex. This has confused me! Do books involving a mother and father educate children about heterosexual sex?

There is also a ban on gay marriages here in Australia and that shows us that homophobia is here in this country. I don't know how we are going to be protected by the law here in Australia. I'm certainly not protected by the law in Muslim countries. It seems discriminatory to me. Religious teachings include stories of conquering and bloody wars. I don't understand why certain religious leaders wish to prevent the teaching of inclusion and love. When suicide is so common in the queer community, it can never be too early to teach acceptance.

I get the sense that children learn about the world through the stories they're exposed to, so books like the one you mention sound like a wonderful way to introduce them to same-sex relationships and diverse sorts of families. I suppose a question you are asking is: 'What does it mean when religious and political leaders do not take up responsibility to promote and encourage acceptance?'

Yeah, and these views seem to 'win the game' – they become a taken-for-granted 'truth' in society. That's a sad state of affairs.

We have previously talked about the challenges of 'coming out' and how this concept did not fit for you. Through our conversations you described the art of inviting people to 'come in' to your life. How have you been able to explore alternative and preferred ways of being when the games of truth try to dominate? What does this action say about the hopes you have for your life?

Well, when I started to visit gay organisations, some would prescribe to me how I should 'come out' and then let my entire extended family deal with this. They would say, 'To tell people is to say you're proud of who you are' or that I wouldn't be able to be a fully happy person if I didn't 'come out' in particular ways. They would say simply, 'People need to deal with it and get over it'. I felt some sort of pressure to make my sexuality public.

This didn't seem quite so straightforward to me. Perhaps it was because I am really proud of who I am, and I feel like I am a fully happy person, that I was able to look at other ways of living my life. I know that if I had the choice to be straight, I wouldn't choose it. Even if I don't tell certain members of my extended family about my sexuality, I don't view myself as in the closet, in a dark place that I must escape from. Far from it, this 'closet' is full of precious things, like things you could never afford to buy! It's my treasure chest. The way I see it, rather than me needing to move out of the closet, to make my sexuality public to everyone, including my grandparents, instead I get to choose who to open the door to, and who to invite to 'come in' to my life.

This different metaphor took away the pressure I had been feeling. I no longer feel a pressure to 'come out' to my entire family, and instead I have many precious people who I have invited to 'come in' to my life. I am hoping that other people in my situation don't feel the pressure of these 'games of truth' to make a public move that doesn't fit for them. I like the fact that I choose people to 'come in' to my life. Importantly, I choose people who I think are valuable to support me and share things that are important to me.

Can you tell me how you have experimented with this 'coming in' idea?

Well yes. Once I started to think of inviting specific people to 'come in', rather than me 'coming out', I found it easier to think of ways to invite my mum, dad, and siblings into my life ... into my treasure chest. I wanted to share my jewels! I remember the day vividly. You and I talked about it together first and prepared a 'first aid kit'. We came up with some good plans.

Plan One: I took my family to a café, a public space. Plan Two: I said to them that I loved them dearly and I wanted them to be part of my life. I said that what I was going to tell them was to make it possible for them to come in to my life. When I said: 'I am gay and can never imagine being with a woman', Mum began to cry and said at first, 'Why are you doing this to me?'. My dad did not say a word. I could understand my mother was in pain and she needed time. But she is happy for me now. She has invited me and my boyfriend to dinner. She still worries about what Allah might do to me. The other day it was so cute when she said to me, 'Son, I love you and I will not let Allah put you in hell. I will stand before him and say you created my son'. She also tells my sisters to tell me to wear a condom!

My sisters are so accepting; they were like ... 'Why has it taken you so long to tell us?' But my brother – sorry Hassan – that's a different story. He fights with all of us. I know he means well, but he doesn't get it. He reckons if I go to the mosque, or pay for therapy, or be given some male hormone, then I will stop being such a queen and instead be a man. Hassan says he understands I'm gay, somehow different from him, because he could never imagine being able to root a bloke, but he says I should stay celibate to avoid going to hell. Dad's still is a bit quiet. He needs more time.

How are you able to hold on to this idea of inviting people to 'come in' to your life despite what you were up against?

I've been up against heaps of things: the attitudes of some people in the Muslim faith, the gay community about needing to 'come out', and then the political issues. I think I have become good friends with silence.

I'm interested in this friendship with silence. I have heard an idea about friendships with silence. Would you be interested in hearing about this?

Yep, that's okay.

According to the therapist, Johnella Bird, silence is sometimes a resource for people to use to survive. So, instead of people being silenced, they take up the silence when they need to. Does this idea resonate for you?

Mmm … It's definitely an action I use to ignore the bullshit I hear.

So it is something you take up … is its presence helpful?

Well yeah, it's like a loyal and reliable mate. It can help you get through the tough times. It keeps me sane. And it helps me … it keeps me connected to my faith.

What is it that you hold precious and value about your faith? Why is this important to you?

I have never been asked this question. I suppose some people might think that I would dump my faith because it's not gay-friendly … but that would just be playing into another truth game! I suppose my faith is important to me because it reminds me … it keeps me close to my family and the memories.

What do you mean by the memories?

I used to love particular times we spent as a family. We would sit around our father while he would tell us stories about the Prophets. He would tell stories about how the Prophet advocated for women's rights at a time when they were being buried at birth, and how the Prophet didn't discriminate against colour. It was a black man, Bilal, who led the prayers in ancient times. I also love what Islam means, and that is peace.

Of course, Islam, like most religions, has its issues with sexuality. In some Muslim countries, we hear of honour killings and violence against gay people. These may have more to do with cultural beliefs, rather than Quranic, but I'm not sure if this is much comfort to Muslim women or gay people! In my experience, within the Muslim community there is interest in questioning Islamophobic rhetoric, but less interest in dealing with the political and human rights violations suffered by women or gay people.

Who else knows what you're up against?

I hope my family. I know my sisters do and other Muslim gay people, maybe.

What might they appreciate in the steps that you took to tell your story?

They know that I'm taking a big risk, but I know that it's important to tell my story because I'm challenging the thoughts of the gay community about coming out. I'm wanting to live a gay life but to keep my faith and stay linked to my society in general. It's a triple whammy, to be gay, Arab, and Muslim.

What might you contribute to other people in similar circumstances as yourself?

I hope I contribute to the sense that you can be whoever you want to be.

A Definitional Ceremony

Definitional ceremonies (Russell and Carey, 2004; White, 2000) provide a therapeutic arena for the performance of the preferred narratives of people's lives, identities, and relationships. In this therapeutic arena, Jamil invited his brother to witness a performance of the stories of his life. Hassan then had the opportunity to respond to these tellings by re-telling certain aspects of the conversation that resonated a fascination or new understanding for him. Hassan was invited to swap chair positions with Jamil. The questions that I asked Hassan were guided by a map that consists of four specific categories of inquiry (White, 2000). These four categories included:

1. Identifying certain expressions spoken by Jamil: Hassan was asked to reflect on what particular expressions from Jamil's stories struck a chord for him.
2. Describing the image: Hassan was asked to speak about what images of Jamil's life, of his identities, and journey, were evoked for Hassan as he listened to his brother.

3. Embodying responses: Hassan engaged in a process of exploring the aspects of his own experiences of life that resonated with these expressions, and with the images evoked by these expressions.
4. Acknowledging transport: In this concluding part of the process, Hassan was invited to reflect on how he was moved on account of being present to witness Jamil's expressions of his life.

The transcript below highlights the powerfully moving re-tellings that Hassan offered. In this process, Hassan was able to reflect on Jamil's preferred claims about his life and his identities. His brother's story became more visible to him, and there was an opportunity to articulate shared themes and values. This therapeutic arena provided a forum for these two brothers to acknowledge a different awareness of each other's lives, which may not have otherwise been possible.

Identifying the expression: *As you listened to Jamil's story, which expressions caught your attention?*

It's my brother ... Oh man, I didn't ... I didn't realise why he told us, why he put it out there ... it was not to shock me ... he chose to tell me because he wanted me to 'come in' to his life. I thought he just wanted to piss me off.

Describing the image: *What did this suggest to you about Jamil's purposes, values, beliefs, hopes, dreams, and commitments?*

I heard that he just wants to be accepted and respected for who he is, but everything around him rejects him and I have been guilty of that. I thought he gave up his faith and I'm scared for him because I don't want him to go to hell. I feel like it's my duty to protect him as his brother. I didn't realise how hard it was for him.

Embodying responses: *What is it about your life that accounts for why these expressions caught your attention or struck a chord for you?*

Well it's pretty tough for me being a Muslim with all the media hype about terrorists, wars, and rapists. I've wanted to change my name because, as soon as they think you're Muslim, people treat you like ... well they all get paranoid. But I can go to the Mosque and I'm accepted. But where can Jamil go? It must be even tougher if you add being gay to being an Arab and Muslim.

Acknowledging transport: *Where has this experience taken you to, that you would not otherwise have arrived at, if you hadn't been present as an audience to this conversation?*

I didn't realise how tough it was for him. I never have thought about what society says about the gay community, about how much he has had to go through. I just thought that gays are accepted in the west ... I didn't think of the politics and all the other stuff. Anyway, it makes me think, if you knew the consequence would be death or hell, why would you choose it? It's still hard for me to get my head around it because I'm a bit confused. Why would he choose it? It's hard to think something different to what you've been taught. I heard a quote from the Quran that 'Allah made us all different so that we can learn from one another'. I don't know ... I think this message needs to be spread.

That's a powerful quote, if people were able to hold this quote in their lives, what might be different?

I think people hear what they want to hear. Words are different to the practice.

Well, sitting here today to hear your brother's story, what does this practice speak to you of?

Loyalty.

At this point, Hassan put his head down and began to sob. No further words were said, but the tears spoke. They spoke to me of a bond of the womb, an honouring of two brothers' relationship. This honouring may have never appeared if certainty had taken me over, or if the 'games of truth' had not been exposed. The brothers embraced and I shed tears too.

Reflections on this Process

To me, this process reflects the importance of Foucault's (2003b, 173) descriptions of making conflicts more visible:

> It is a matter of making conflicts more visible of making them more essential than mere clashes of interest or mere institutional blockages. From the conflicts and clashes a new relation of forces must emerge whose temporary profile will be a reform.

In this instance, the conflict seemed to lie in Hassan's perception of Jamil's sexuality as opposing his values; however, this conflict was exposed and the definitional ceremony provided an opportunity for both brothers to speak more richly of what was important to them. A performance then took place that led to a re-definition of loyalty. It was loyalty that had brought Hassan to come to listen to his brother's story. It was loyalty that shaped his responses. And, by the end of this conversation, both brothers were leaving with a much richer appreciation of what loyalty meant to them, and what it would make possible in their relationship.

To make this performance possible, the stage had to be set in a particular way – the conversation had to be scaffolded. The backdrop was a deconstruction of certain 'games of truth', including the dominant cultural ideas about homosexuality and 'queerying' the concept of coming out. Exploring the art of resistance was also significant. Enquiries into Jamil's intentions and hopes led to richer descriptions and explanations of why he was living his life in certain ways. Then, and only then, did Hassan have the chance to join the stories of his life with those of his brother. The categories of questions allowed Hassan to respond in ways that resonated with his brother. Once the stage had been set, the performance took place. It was a performance of honesty, of brotherhood, and of loyalty. And from within their shared faith emerged a significant shared value: 'Allah made us all different so that we can learn from one another'. As a woman from a Muslim heritage, I hope this chapter has unveiled some of the pertinent issues that exist within Muslim GLBTIQ communities. I have been privileged to work in collaboration within these communities and witness the performances of different meanings of self, alternative stories of life, and the generation of new possibilities for relationship. Exploring issues of sexuality in the therapeutic realm can be challenging, but in the process I have been invited to 'come in' to an amazing learning journey about people's knowledges and skills in the realm of sexuality, society, spirituality, and religion.

Acknowledgements

I am grateful to Jamil and Hassan for granting me the permission to share their story. I would like to honour Jamil's and Hassan's courage, strength, and resilience in their attempts to develop a connection, and share their stories in the midst of the current climate affecting Arab Muslims. I'd also like to acknowledge David Denborough's encouragement to use the written word to make more visible the complexities of sexual, religious and cultural identities. I forward a special thank you to the staff at the Dulwich Centre, The Corner Youth Health Service, Charing Cross Narrative Centre, and Macquarie University, who stimulate and support my passion for engaging with narrative ideas. I also express gratitude to the reviewers for indulging me in their thought provoking comments and invaluable contributions. Finally, I give thanks to Lynz for inspiring this book and supporting practitioners to *queery* the dilemmas in therapy.

References

Amundson, J. Stewart, K. and Valentine, L. (1993), Temptations of power and certainty. *Journal of Marital and Family Therapy*, 19(2): 111–123.
Bird, J. (2000), *The Heart's Narrative* (Edge Press: Auckland).

Foucault, M. (2003a), The ethics of the concern of the self as a practice of freedom. In P. Rabinow, and N. Rose (eds), *The Essential Foucault*, 25–43 (New York: The News Press).

Foucault, M. (2003b), 'So is it important to think?' In P. Rabinow and N. Rose (eds), *The Essential Foucault*, 170–174 (New York: The News Press).

Gay and Lesbian Counselling and Community Services of Australia (n.d.), *Coming Out*. Retrieved 5 August 2006, from <http:/www.glccs.org.au/coming_out. html>.

Harding, B. and Harding, V. (2002), *The Rainbow Cubby House* (Sydney: Bulldog Books).

Manji, I. (2003), *The Trouble with Islam* (Sydney: Random House).

Mears, B. (2002), 'Lee's acts of resistance', *Narrative Network News*, December: 5.

Myerhoff, B. (1982), Life history among the elderly: Performance, visibility and remembering. In J. Ruby (ed.), *A Crack in the Mirror: Reflexive Perspectives in Anthropology*, 99–117 (Philadelphia: University of Pennsylvania Press).

Nicholas, J. and Howard, J. (1998), Better dead than gay? *Youth Studies Australia*, 17(4): 28–33.

Russell, S. and Carey. M. (2004), *Narrative Therapy: Responding to Your Questions* (Adelaide: Dulwich Centre Publications).

Vygotsky, L. (1986), *Thought and Language* (Cambridge: MIT Press).

Wade, A. (1997), Small acts of living: Everyday resistance to violence and other forms of oppression. *Contemporary Family Therapy*, 19: 23–39.

Woodcock, S. (2004), Globalisation of LGBT identities: Containment masquerading as salvation or why lesbians have less fun. In M. Frunza and T. Vacarescu (eds), *Gender and the (Post) East-West Divide*, 1–13, Retrieved 5 February 2007, from <http://www.iiav.nl/epublications/2005/gendeRomania.pdf>.

White, M. and Epston, D. (1990), *Narrative Means to Therapeutic Ends* (New York: W.W. Norton).

White, M. (1995), *Re-authoring Lives: Interviews and Essays* (Adelaide: Dulwich Centre Publications).

White, M. (2000), Reflecting-team work as definitional ceremony revisited. In M. White, *Reflections on Narrative Practice: Essays and Interviews*, 59–85 (Adelaide: Dulwich Centre Publications).

White, M. (2006). Narrative practice with families with children: Externalising conversations revisited. In M. White and A. Morgan, *Narrative Therapy with Children and Their Families*, 1–56 (Adelaide: Dulwich Centre Publications).

Websites about Queer, Arab, and Muslim Issues

Al Fatiha Foundation <www.al-fatiha.org>. A North American organisation for gay and lesbian Muslims.

GayMiddleEast.com contains interesting and helpful country by-country information with recent gay-related news reports.

Huriyah: A Queer Muslim Magazine <www.huriyahmag.com>. An on-line magazine for Queer Muslims.

Queer Jihad <www.well.com/user/queerjhd/index.htm>. According to this site, 'Queer Jihad is the queer Muslim struggle for acceptance: first, the struggle to accept ourselves as being exactly the way Allah has created us to be; and secondly, the struggle for understanding among Muslims in general'.

The Gay and Lesbian Arabic Society (GLAS) <www.glas.org>. An international organisation established in the USA in 1988 with worldwide chapters, GLAS serves as a networking organisation for Gays and Lesbians of Arab descent or those living in Arab countries.

Chapter 11

Cultural Competence with BDSM Lifestyles

Dossie Easton

The sources of information in this chapter include 20 years experience providing therapy for Bondage, Discipline, Sadism and Masochism (BDSM) practitioners and 35 years of personal experience of the leather communities working as an educator and learning from my own experiences, from my colleagues and friends, and, most importantly, from my clients, to whom I am most grateful for sharing the intimate truths of their lives and their ways of loving in therapy. In this chapter I will share information, ideas and some speculation on psychodynamic theory about doing therapy with individuals and partnerships involved in sado-masochistic or S/M lifestyles. If you are a therapist seeking to understand and learn about BDSM practice, I applaud you. Too many professionals believe that they know all they need to know about how BDSM is practiced and who wants to do it. Everyone seems to believe they have a right to voice their opinions whether or not they have any actual information, and so what the public hears about S/M is often uninformed, misinformed and downright mythological.

The practice of S/M covers such a wide territory that it is just about impossible to define it. S/M is referred to by many names. The currently popular "BDSM" comes from "Bondage and Discipline," "Dominance and Submission," and "Sadism and Masochism." Sometimes it is called "leather" in general, "erotic power play" in particular, or just plain "kink" to denote the unusual and explorative nature of these sexual practices. The participants often refer to themselves as "players." The territory may include: uncommon sexual practices, bondage and helplessness, intense and unusual stimulations, erotic role play, service and submission, fetishes, and much more. One writer has defined S/M with admirably concise wit as: "Power games for fun rather than profit."

It is important for the therapist to understand that for most people, S/M is not only a sexual practice but a way of life. The S/M communities have developed a widespread culture of their own, complete with art, literature, theater, support organizations, meeting places, spiritual practice, conferences, and other gatherings. The culture explores, supports and develops radically new expressions of sexuality that expand our understanding of sex, relationship and humanity, based on experiences that often contradict assumptions of the mainstream culture and established paradigms of sexuality, relationship and psychodynamics. The therapist working with BDSM clients will need to acquire some knowledge of the communities in which their clients live and build families, and a respect for this evolving culture. Since it is possible to live almost entirely within the leather communities, S/M knowledge and awareness may permeate all aspects of a client's life, and familiarity with role play, fantasy, mythos and power dynamics may show up in areas of therapy that have nothing to do with sex. We are talking about BDSM practice that is safe, sane and consensual. I assume the reader knows that this is possible, and does not need me to point out that careful, thoughtful, highly functional people have been enjoying these practices for a long time with no negative consequences.[1] The therapist seeking to know more about these cultures should definitely read some of the books written by BDSM practitioners to learn about how S/M people negotiate consent and insure safety while exploring at the outer limits of what "erotic" might contain. A reading list is provided at the end of this article.

Given the enormous range of possibilities, and that the practices in a particular individual's lifestyle will most often change and evolve over time, what does the therapist need to know to consider themselves culturally competent to work with a client in these often mythologized and pathologized relationships?

Comfort Level

The first thing you need to know is yourself. To be a good therapist you must look at your own comfort level in dealing with BDSM, and be prepared to be honest with clients about your experience and beliefs. This writer had an interesting experience as a client with a therapist who was not accustomed to any form of self-disclosure. When I asked her what her opinions of S/M were, she dodged. I said I needed to hear something from her to feel safe; she said she would think about it. The next week she came in and talked to me about her understandings: that S/M was much maligned, that it was obvious that healthy people did it, that it was present in many aspects of our culture, as evidenced by the popularity of scary movies. That was enough to reassure me that she would not pathologize me—we worked together for more than five years, and I credit her with being the best therapist I have ever worked with. Reading can offer you not only information but also the opportunity to check where you are comfortable and, perhaps more important, what pushes your buttons. No need to condemn yourself here, no one expects you to have no reactions at all. Your most important task is to be aware of your hot buttons, and take them into account when working with your clients. Only then can you be truly present to hold the space in therapy in a welcoming and supportive manner.

Knowing your own buttons helps you to decide whether or not you might choose to work with a particular client. I have referred one client whose fantasies, often expressed with a lot of rage, were leaving me feeling lost and frightened. After trying various techniques to calm myself and get present with his fantasies,

---

1   People from all walks of life use or define as BDSM. This even includes psychologists, academics and therapists. See the well written *Safe, Sane and Consensual: Contemporary Perspectives on Sadomasochism* by Darren Langdridge and Meg Barker, 2008.

and failing, I sent him to another practitioner, where he did well and got his needs met better than he could have with me. That practitioner now refers clients to me, so there has been no loss to my practice, indeed, my practice has been enhanced. So be proud of yourself if, after careful consideration, you decide to refer a client because of your own comfort level. Think of it as networking.

Evaluating a Client

How does a therapist evaluate the sanity and functionality of an S/M person? Exactly as you would anyone else, by how well they function. Does this person have work, friends, family, relationships, the basics of a healthy life? Therapists can easily evaluate functioning no matter how unfamiliar they may be with a client's sexuality. When meeting a new client, particularly one new to BDSM, I also evaluate their sources of information and their connections to community. Has this person read any of the good books, or do they follow discussions online? BDSM community has developed enormously within the last 20 or 30 years, and this once utterly secret underground now has a rich literature and access to many support groups, gatherings, play spaces, and educational opportunities. When a person gets together with other players on a regular basis to share information and experiences, their practice is much better informed and more secure. On the other hand, a person who is isolated or only connected through the internet can make mistakes through isolation or lack of accurate information. We will discuss the rich communities that are available to your clients, and where a client might start to access them, further on. Serious questions may arise when a client is a survivor of child abuse, and you hear some similarities between his or her S/M fantasies and actual historical trauma. I do not believe that trauma survivors are of necessarily automata doomed by childhood experiences to continue to seek out what has harmed them because they don't know any better and can't make other choices. What I believe, following my own experience and observations, is that we all tend to be attracted to opportunities to relive some of our painful history because we have a healthy desire to struggle with these issues and empower ourselves by working toward a better outcome.

S/M can be an excellent venue for that struggle, since it occurs in a particularly boundaried area of a person's life, and the person is free to write the script, add new elements such as respect for limits, boundaries and personhood, and transform the denouement into a scenario of desire and delight and love. S/M is not therapy, but it can contribute a great deal to the therapeutic process.

Scene Space

Crucial to understanding the nature of S/M as it is practiced today is the notion of scene space. BDSM is often described in theatrical terms: a session is a scene, the people who do it are players, they may be playing roles, they may be following a script, the bedroom may become the playroom. This language reinforces the truth that the roles that we play in S/M are most often very different from the roles a person may play at work or school or any other part of their lives. Scene space denotes the ways in which the reality inhabited in the course of enacting an S/M fantasy is different and separate from the reality that may be inhabited the rest of the time. Scene space is a subjective boundary that sets apart S/M experience from day to day living.

Scene space is a protected space, in which the players agree to generate whatever safety is needed to take the risks and open up the vulnerabilities that are so important to successful S/M play. It is considered all-important to enter into scene space as into a sacred space, with carefully negotiated interdependence, in which the participants count on each other to remain open and exquisitely sensitive to each others' needs, in which they agree to respect each others' limits and boundaries without fail, in which they promise to stay highly conscious and to support each others' journeys into the outer reaches of their personal possibilities. In scene space, players must be safe to drop conventional boundaries and enter into intense vulnerabilities.

In scene space players become free to be both larger than life and to be terribly small. They are free to try on roles, try out personae, be the wild person they never thought they could be, or the accomplished sexual athlete of their dreams. Some role play explorations can be downright silly, and lots of fun—in that scary dungeon, you may see people laughing and shrieking, clowning sometimes, right in the middle of sex. You may see people cowering and weeping, or towering and threatening, or leering like the best of vampires in beloved gothic novels. Scene space is a wildlife sanctuary for everyone's precious inner wilderness.

Some Myths

There are a lot of myths about BDSM and the people who participate in it—too many to cover, much less respond to, in this article.[2] The most all-consuming stereotype is that S/M players are all self or other destructive, perhaps "unconsciously," and are enacting hidden agendas that will inevitably cause them and their lovers severe psychological, if not physical, damage. A look at the actual people who practice BDSM will show you a group of almost spectacularly functional souls: many professionals, long term marriages, parents—whatever criteria of high functioning human you ascribe to, you will find them in the S/M community. That does not mean that S/M communities are any freer from the scourges of abuse, domestic violence, enmeshed relationships and emotional bullying than any other group of people, but such problems afflict only a minority, as they do in the rest of the culture.

---

2   For a fuller discussion of myths and stereotypes, read Langdridge and Barker, 2008.

It is particularly enlightening to realize, for instance if you were to attend a support group meeting or an S/M class, that many of BDSM's community leaders and most powerful and contributing members are, in fact, bottoms or submissives in their play, although often quite different in the rest of their lives. In their everyday lives they may be doctors, lawyers, teachers, even therapists. Such community leaders are affectionately known as "alpha bottoms." The people who identify as dominant are often sweet, courteous, quiet, perhaps even little shy. They only act like villains if you ask them very nicely.

Another common myth about S/M is that fantasies and fetishes limit the individual who acts on them in the sense that they will not be able to enjoy sex or orgasm without satisfying their very particular kink. It is just about never true that a player becomes impotent without their fetish. Some people new to the scene start out focused on a particular fantasy, often a cherished and richly embroidered bedtime story that they seek to bring into reality, and don't see themselves as trying anything else. But, when they find a partner who is happy to explore their beloved script with the attention to detail that years of dreaming can develop, they may also find that that partner has fantasies of their own that they would like to enact, and the erstwhile single-minded fetishist almost immediately starts building a rich repertoire (or losing partners at an overly rapid rate). Then perhaps the two of them will read a story about another fantasy or observe someone else's adventure at a play party and be inspired to try *that* and thus the new explorer will find their repertoire expanding to unexpected richness far beyond the boundaries of any initial fixation.

Safety

BDSM players place great importance on safety, and learning what they need to know before trying to operate, say, a cane or a bondage position. Community connections, classes and good reading are seen as obviously necessary, just as one might seek out a class or a manual before participating in any strenuous sport. The internet offers no guarantees of accuracy, so information and ideas gleaned from the web must be received with caution and confirmed with further checking. My experience is that my judgment is keener when I see and hear the person imparting information, so I prefer to attend classes in person.

One couple who consulted with me because their attempts to play with bondage had not worked had been trying to learn how from the internet. When I recommended some workshops where they could learn in person about how to do what they both desired to do, they felt they could never expose their kink to other people, not even other kinksters. They showed me a photograph of a bondage position they had tried to reproduce: when I looked at it, I realized that the bondage in the picture would never work in the real world—it had been "Photoshopped."

Consent

S/M players most often establish safewords—agreed upon code words that allow someone to interrupt a scene to take care of something that isn't working well without dropping out of their role. Safewords may be designed to use as communication when a scene is scripted on make-believe nonconsent, as many fantasies are: some players delight in moaning "No, no, no," when they would be very disappointed if their partner were to stop. Commonly used safewords are "Red", which means "Stop we need to talk"; "Yellow," which means "Lighten up, please," or "You're way ahead of me"; and "Green," which means "This is great you could go faster/harder/deeper and I would love it a lot." I like to emphasize to my clients that when someone uses a safeword, we should assume that both the safeworder and their partner are in a particularly vulnerable moment, and the appropriate response is to move into a modality of mutual support. I make a point of teaching my clients that interrupting a scene to deal with a problem is a valuable skill, especially as they become adept at recovering their place in the scene and resuming their play after taking care of whatever problem had occurred.

Thoughtful S/M practitioners place very high value on informed consent and often spend a great deal of time considering what might be included in a scene and what would be outside their limits. Negotiation is particularly important when the territory can include flogging, piercing, scarification, and an enormous range of intense stimulations. Sometimes participants write their limits down to make sure everyone is on the same page. Conversely, if a client tells you that consent isn't important or is only for sissies, you might wonder about the safety of their practice.

We are often asked how to distinguish consensual BDSM from abuse. Informed consent is obviously the first criterion, and I like to use a slightly expanded definition of consent. I understand consent to be an active collaboration between all persons involved in any interaction, for the pleasure and benefit of all. This rules out bullying, emotional blackmail, pushing limits without consent, and all forms of exploitation. Sometimes you can judge by the results; everyone should feel better off and better about themselves after good scene.

Communities

I use this word in the plural because there are so many different groups and identities within the larger umbrella of "people into BDSM." Some communities are defined by their members: women, men, lesbian, gay, bisexual, straight, and so on, while others define themselves by their practices: dominance and submission, bondage, sadism and masochism, fantasy role play and the like. Many community events are open to all of the above, others specialize—which they will tell you about in their invitations and advertisements. There is a growing movement called TNG for The Next Generation of younger players who bring their own perspectives which are always very interesting to me, since these players got to come out into S/M supported by the enormously expanded resources of community, information, and permission.

One easy way to connect to any local community is to search online for a "munch" in your area. Munches are weekly or monthly meetings, usually held in restaurants that have a back room that can be reserved for the purpose, where people who may know each other from online discussion groups get together in person to eat a meal together, get to know each other, and talk, talk, talk. A person thinking about entering the leather community can go to a munch in ordinary clothes and see what the characters in their fantasies actually look like in their everyday personae.

In many urban communities, there are "play party" spaces, sometimes called dungeons, where people can go to an invitation only party and play on large equipment—sort of like jungle gyms and swings for grown ups -that they may not be able to afford or fit in their homes. These parties can represent a safe space to explore play with a new partner, or new stimulations, surrounded by knowledgeable and like-minded people who can help out if anything goes awry. Dungeons often become community centers, hosting everything from leather-friendly 12-step meetings to knitting circles, and sponsoring classes on weekday evenings and weekend afternoons where experienced players teach the technical details of S/M practices.

These workshops are well attended, not only to acquire necessary and useful information, but also because an individual who shows up at classes demonstrates an attitude of responsibility toward learning how to enact their fantasies safely, which is well respected in this community. BDSM classes offer a good environment in which to meet other players and make friends, free of the pressures of cruising. I often advise clients new to the community to attend a workshop with the intention, not of hunting for the partner of their dreams, but of meeting someone like themselves, that they can be friends with and learn from.

Many urban areas have developed S/M support groups—the San Francisco Bay Area where I live boasts quite a few of them—that a client can join to make friends, get support, and learn how to operate both their toy collections and their fantasies. Most groups meet once a month for discussion, a speaker or an educational demonstration. Local support groups can usually be found on line.

You Already Have Many Skills

The therapist who wants further reassurance about safety can always ask a respectful question. I recall a client who told me that her play with her partner wasn't safe, and I asked what he had done that concerned her. She told me he had put her into a bathtub with a 12-volt car battery. (Every time I have told this story to a BDSM audience, the room has gone silent here—you can practically hear the shock.) Firmly letting go of my own ideas about what is and is not safe, I asked her if she thought that was safe: she said no. No physical harm had actually occurred, and my client and I now had agreement that we could work on what she felt was unsafe.

A therapist can ask a client how the client ensures safety with a particular practice—asking a respectful question is always all right, but please don't assume that you know the answer. Your client may be the expert on their practices. Injuries caused by S/M are uncommon; the practice has a much higher safety rating than, for one example, skiing.

This being said, most people from the leather communities come to therapists to work on the same issues anyone else would: for help in their struggle with anxiety, depression, conflict and the like. They are fine with any therapist who can hear about their lifestyle without judging or pathologizing. Too often I get "refugees" from therapists who told their clients, often in an initial session, that their lifestyle was their problem. Do they really believe that giving up an unusual sexuality will help a person deal with crushing anxieties about a job search? So the first thing a therapist can do is, again, read some books written by members of the S/M community, a few of which are listed at the end of this article. That way we, as therapists, can deal with our judgments and any of our buttons that might get pushed long before we are sitting in a room with a client who is counting on us to treat them with respect and positive regard.

To approach clients in a nonjudgmental stance requires not only refraining from pathologizing, but also becoming able to hear and appreciate positive contributions of S/M to a client's life. Clients will need the space to express happiness about new successes in their relationships, and new discoveries in their sexual interactions.

BDSM Issues

Some clients want to work on issues that involve BDSM directly, and this requires more expertise from the therapist. For instance, how does one find a compatible partner? How does one communicate one's desires? How does one check out a potential partner? How does one bring fantasies into reality? Clients seeking support in their initial explorations of these practices will have a lot of questions about how to make things work, how to negotiate, how to operate a toy safely, and how to meet a compatible partner, of which the inexperienced therapist would have little knowledge. Coming out to themselves as an S/M person can be a big challenge to some, and coming out to family and friends is a further, sometimes dangerous project. Some players suffer from growing resentment of the parts of their lives where it is necessary to maintain a "closet" or total secrecy about their lifestyle, their relationships, and their happiness. All of these and more can show up in the therapist's office as a clients goals for therapy. To support a client in these types of goals the therapist will need to be well-informed about how BDSM lifestyles work, and how successful members achieve their desired goals. Some clients come into therapy because their S/M explorations have opened up previously buried experiences of trauma, abuse, or other major emotional conflict.

Journeys in S/M Role Play

S/M role play can become a profound psychological journey into Jungian Shadow territory, as people inhabit roles of victim and villain, child and nurturer, slave and cruel owner. How do people negotiate emotional boundaries in these deep journeys? Who are we when we bring forth our precious inner victim or precious inner bully for an evening of erotic play? Some therapists will be able to follow these processes much like understanding psychodrama, others will have a harder time.

Playing out a dark fantasy may have led the client into some previously split off part of themselves. That makes the S/M play itself valuable as the gateway to a previously inaccessible gestalt of experience, self-concept and, most importantly, split off emotions. Landing right in the middle of one's Shadow can also make the journey pretty scary.

I recall the case of a client, an experienced S/M player, who came into therapy after her initial explorations of role playing "Girl" to her partner's "Daddy" had opened up some intense and powerful inner gestalts. Initially she wondered why she was so obsessively attracted to this partner and the play they shared, as they had very little else in common. It was obvious to her that some very deep drive was finding satisfaction in this form of play, and we looked at how these experiences were awakening a particular form of wounded inner child. The client herself was a survivor of physical abuse from her actual father in her actual childhood.

The relationship continued passionately onward for about three months, when "Daddy" suddenly announced that she had found a primary partner and that "Daddy" was no longer allowed to play with her "Girl." My client fell into a terrible grief. She couldn't sleep, couldn't eat, could barely keep going to her job, and reported that she came home from work every day and fell on the floor crying, "She said she wanted us! Daddy wanted us!" After a couple of months of deep therapy but little respite and increasing exhaustion, my client took a tricyclic antidepressant for about three months.

The progress of her therapy was intense and rewarding. She did a great deal of inner child work, and became able to access the particular part of her that was so severely wounded from the abuse and hear what that child had to say. We were both horrified to hear that this inner child believed that her family would be better off if she were dead or gone away, since they seemed to have so much trouble with her and she was a bad girl who deserved too much punishment. The therapy became focused on nurturance and self-soothing; it seemed important that the client herself take over the job of reparative parenting to her wounded inner child, with myself as therapist serving as transitional support system. This worked, and my client became able to comfort her grieving self so well that she no longer needed the antidepressant. She emerged from this journey stating firmly that she was utterly grateful to have learned what she learned and to have developed an ongoing relationship with her inner child that allowed not only healing but freed her to go to graduate school and reach out for her life goals as she had never dared to do before.

Issues of Identity

Clearly, these deep emotional journeys can bring up many questions about negotiation, boundaries, consent, and trust. People may open up issues of identity—am I truly a slave? A real submissive? Do I have the heart of a dominant? Who am I that I enjoy pretending to be a bully? I take a Jungian point of view here, and look at the various parts we play in the theater of S/M as personae— valid parts of the person, but often minority parts. Where S/M can be healing practice lies in the potential for parts of us that couldn't really exist outside of the negotiated co-dependence of scene space to come into play for an evening, in a loving and consensual relationship; we can get to see ourselves in very new mirrors. Some people live their S/M roles full time, others move in and out of them. Some play many roles, others just one that they see as their core identity. Some confine their role playing to the bedroom, and others live their S/M roles everyday, 24/7. Therapists need to be wary of our culture's love of classification here. Some people believe that people can be classified into groups, perhaps by some trait encoded in the DNA, like gay or straight or male or female or dominant or submissive or S/M or vanilla. Your beliefs about what groups you belong in may be challenged by people whose sexuality is extensively different from your own. Please learn to regard the full range of sexual behavior as part of the birth right of every human being; no one is incapable of acting outside their current definitions of their sexuality. A liberated sexuality may evolve and grow in many ways during an individual's lifetime. Do be cautious about how your clients tend to classify themselves. Our culture is all too supportive of pigeonholing people, and of labeling some of the pigeonholes as pathologies. Individuals exploring a new identity often pigeonhole and pathologize themselves, and cut themselves off from a world of possibility while they define themselves as not okay. The therapist can support the client in maintaining an open mind and a non-judgmental stance about themselves.

Countertransference

How can you, the therapist, take care of yourself when a client's sexual lifestyle gives you the jitters? Reassure yourself that your own sexual choices are just fine, and give yourself permission to not want to do whatever it is that you don't want to do. Not choosing to participate in any activity is a personal prerogative, and it doesn't mean that you are inhibited, uptight, unhip, or in any way lacking. When you feel okay about being yourself, with your own fabulous and rewarding sex life, you will be more able to support your clients in feeling good about being themselves.

Remember that fantasies are a lot like myths or fairy tales—I often think of them as personal mythology—and they most often include some fairly universal material about what people might find sexy. Think about the sadomasochistic themes in popular culture: "thriller" movies, sexy villains, monsters, the eternally pathetic girl in the white nightie. You may recognize some of your own turn-ons in your clients' fantasies and lifestyle choices, and this might push some fairly profound buttons for you. I think it is helpful to recognize that all of our countertransference may be relevant to the therapeutic journeys we facilitate for our clients, and that clarifying what your fantasies or uneasy feelings may tell you about your client's therapy may deepen and enrich the work you are doing together. We as therapists need to be willing to have a little humility: we are not "above it all", we are in it, with our clients, and we will often awaken feelings from our own Shadows. Sometimes your S/M clients may stimulate something that is important to your personal journey. When that is the case, bring up these issues in your own therapy, and learn what gift there may be for you in further investigation into your Shadow.

Treatment Choices

When you as a therapist are confronted with client issues that are so far outside your experience that you question your ability to work with them, you have several choices. Do remember that in depth knowledge about S/M practices can often only be gained by direct experience, which you (quite understandably) might not be interested in acquiring. *Kink Aware Professionals* is an important web site offered by the National Coalition for Sexual Freedom in the US that lists S/M knowledgeable therapists and other professionals (doctors, lawyers and such) by geographical area, so you can always know who the local experts are. When you are concerned about your expertise with a particular client, and reading has not given you the answers you seek, you can ask one of these professionals for a consultation to help you understand and work better with your client—such a consultation is depicted in the useful film from CARAS listed in the reading list. In some cases, it may be appropriate to refer a particular client to a BDSM-qualified professional, just as you might any other client whose concerns you feel not best qualified to address. This is very similar to finding a therapist who speaks, say, Polish, for a client whose English is not fluent enough to support easy communication in therapy.

Shadowplay

I have previously published an article entitled *Shadowplay: S/M Journeys to Our Selves*,[3] in which I explicate in full my understanding of S/M role play as journeys into the personal Shadow that can bring previously forbidden emotions, gestalts, and split off parts of the self into consciousness, somewhat as dreams, fantasies and desires may function as signposts to previously buried material that is ready to be welcomed into the light of awareness. Exploring the darker side of Shadow wisdom can allow a person to integrate their most conflictual facets into one coherent jewel of a self.

S/M role play offers opportunities to try on forbidden fantasies like costumes, to travel into the deep woods of Shadow with a trusted comrade, and to choose, consciously, the destination and denouement of the psychodrama. Role players may choose to enter into these journeys by evoking fear and other difficult emotions, and to complete them by sharing sex and orgasm and love with the same partner who so agreeably terrified them. The active partners in these journeys may serve as theater directors, trusted guide, containers, and instigators who function as a mirror in which a person can see their Shadow side, and at the same time be seen as desirable and lovable. The partner in the receptive role offers a very special mirror of erotic and emotional response to the dominant partner that can empower the dominant's journey into treasuring their Shadow self. Partners may choose to complete this mythic journey with an injection of Eros, or Life Force, in the form of orgasm—Nature's best medicine.

S/M as Spiritual Practice

Many S/M adventurers regard their journeys as spiritual practice. My co-author, Hardy and I have written about this at length in our 2004 book, *Radical Ecstasy: S/M Journeys to Transcendence*. Jung, you may recall, located the gateway to what he termed the "Collective Unconscious," or spiritual awareness, at the very bottom of the personal unconscious. So, dark journeys into Shadow can be liminal, can bring the traveler to the threshold of some amazing revelations about themselves, about love, and about spiritual connectedness. This is what S/M explorers have to offer the world: their amazing expertise at seeking out the doorway to the Light in the murkiest depths of our personal swamps.

Suggested Reading

Brame, W., Brame, G. and Jacobs, J. (1996), *Different Loving* (Emeryville, CA: Greenery Press).

---

3   In *Safe, Sane and Consensual*—see Suggested Reading list.

Carrellas, B. (2007), *Urban Tantra* (Emeryville, CA: Greenery Press).

Easton, D. and Hardy, J.W. (2004), *Radical Ecstasy: SM Journeys to Transcendence* (Emeryville, CA: Greenery Press).

Henkin. W. and Holiday, S. (1996), *Consensual Sadomasochism* (Greenery Press).

Langdridge, D. and Barker, M. (eds) (2008), *Safe, Sane and Consensual* (Basingstoke: Palgrave).

Thompson, M. (ed.) (1991), *Leatherfolk* (Emeryville, CA: Greenery Press).

Wiseman, J. (2001), *SM 101* (Emeryville, CA: Greenery Press).

[Video] *CARAS Presents Therapy with BDSM Clients*, Dr. Gabrielle Hoff, videographer <www.LifeStyleEducation.net>, 2008 <www.CARAS.ws>.

Index